real
SAM SABOURA'S
style

SAM SABOURA'S

real

STYLE SECRETS

FOR

real women

WITH

real bodies

style

Sam Saboura

with L. G. Mansfield

Clarkson Potter/Publishers
New York

Copyright © 2005 by SamStyles, Inc.
Illustrations copyright © 2005 by Bunky Hurter

Published in the United States by Clarkson Potter/Publishers, an imprint of
the Crown Publishing Group, a division of Random House, Inc., New York.
www.crownpublishing.com
www.clarksonpotter.com

CLARKSON N. POTTER is a trademark and POTTER and colophon are
registered trademarks of Random House, Inc.

Library of Congress Cataloging-in-Publication Data
Saboura, Sam.
  Sam Saboura's real style : style secrets for real women with real bodies / by
Sam Saboura with L. G. Mansfield.
      p. cm.
  1. Fashion. 2. Women's clothing. 3. Beauty, Personal. 4. Somatotypes. I. Title:
Real style style secrets for real women with real bodies. II. Title: Style secrets for real
women with real bodies. III. Mansfield, L. G. IV. Title.
  TT507.S213 2005
  646'.34—dc22

                                                          2005005353

ISBN 1-4000-9771-1
Printed in the United States

Design by Maggie Hinders

10 9 8 7 6 5 4 3 2 1

First Edition

For my mother, Ilham,
who will always be the epitome of real style in my book

acknowledgments

My thanks begin with Elle Mansfield, my partner in crime (and style), who waved her magic wand over every chapter of this book and helped to create something we could both be proud of. There are not enough cropped, yellow, on-sale, cashmere Fendi sweaters in the world to thank you with, and this experience would be nothing without you. You are truly fabulous.

To Bunky Hurter, whose illustrations brought *Real Style* to life. Your wonderful talent and knowledge of design have been an immense contribution to this book. Thank you.

To my family, who endured my constantly hanging up the phone on them in midsentence and put up with my ranting and screaming while I wrote and wrote. I thank you for your love and support, and for being one of a kind. Mom, Nabil, Bruce, and Irene—I love you guys.

To MB. You are the spine of this book. Your patience is unwavering and unconditional, as is your love. I am eternally grateful for everything always.

To my team of teams—the crème de la crème—I thank you from the bottom of my heart:

- My manager, Craig Dorfman; Alex Hertzberg; and everyone at Blueprint, for talking to me ten times a day, every day, and always making me laugh. "No, Craig, thank you."
- My lawyer, Neal Tabachnick, one of the kindest and most meticulous people I have ever met, and the man who always protects my best interests.
- My agent, Hayden Meyer; Ronak Kordestani; and everyone at United Talent, for your energy, optimism, hustle, and dedication.

- My literary agent, PJ Mark, at Collins McCormick, for bringing me to Clarkson Potter and always reminding me that this is *my* book. My deepest gratitude for this wonderful opportunity and for putting up with my five-minute-long voice-mail messages.
- My publicists at mPRm: Jennifer Rettig, Katie Watson, and Katie Sanseverino. If I were Charlie, you'd be my Angels. Thanks for always making it happen—and kicking ass.
- My styling agent, Jamie Haynes, and everyone at Rouge, for keeping me busy when I was already busy enough. Thanks for being there from the beginning.

Thank you to the folks at Clarkson Potter for giving this book a home and fostering a wonderful and challenging journey for me. I cannot imagine working with anyone else.

- To Natalie Kaire, my editor, for always steering me down the right path and helping me make the right choices when I could not see what they were. You have been patient, understanding, and a pleasure to work with.
- To Marysarah Quinn, creative director, for your inspired input.
- To Chris Pavone, executive editor, Pam Krauss, editorial director, and Lauren Shakely, publisher, for your ardent belief in *Real Style* from day one.
- To Tammy Blake, publicity director, and Melanie DeNardo, publicist, for your continued support and attention to detail for the publicity campaign.
- To Maggie Hinders, senior designer, for your lively enthusiasm and gorgeous design, which have made this book one of a kind.
- To Patty Bozza, production editor, and Alison Forner, production manager, for pulling out all the stops on producing a gorgeous book.
- And to the Crown Publishing Group crew—Tina Constable, publicity director, Philip Patrick, marketing director, and Sydney Webber, Potter marketing director—for your brilliant ideas to get *Real Style* out there.

A special thank you to Rita Rago, my mentor, who changed my life with a single phone call. None of this would have been possible without you and your endless support. Love you, Ri.

To everyone at ABC Television and New Screen Entertainment for the *Extreme Makeover* experience, which has allowed me to write this book. I am forever grateful. Andrea Wong, Chuck Bangert, Lou Gorfain, Hank O'Karma, Julie Laughlin, Janis Biewend, Mozelle Miley, and all the staff and crew at New Screen Entertainment—thanks for everything.

To Julie Cooper, the original founder of "The Fashion Family." You plucked me from obscurity and slapped me on TV, and my head is still spinning. I thank you and love you. "We'll always have Max Nugus!"

To Susan Lawlor, my dear friend and fashion producer. You are crazy and talented—all in one. Thanks for always looking out for me. "Hey?"

Special thanks to Mary Clayton, Mark Muir, Tlaloc Villarreal, and Arundel Bell. You guys are all nuts, by the way, and you thought it was me who's crazy! Thanks for putting up with my BS on a daily basis.

To Andrew Glassman, for putting in a good word at ABC and always supporting me. Many thanks.

To Stuart Krasnow, for bringing me onboard the AJ train. You are a wonderful EP and dear friend. Thanks.

To Ron Herman, for seven priceless years that transformed a boy who thought he knew about fashion and style into a man who could write a book about it. What can I say? They were the best of times. I miss them and I thank you.

To all my dear friends, who remained my friends even while I wrote this book, even when I never returned their phone calls, and even when I blew them off for work. You are the most fashionable and fabulous people I know, and you're a constant source of inspiration—if not headache—for me each and every day. I am nothing without you. You know who you are, so consider yourselves mentioned and get over it. There are way too many names to list, and I would probably screw up the order and piss everyone off (Juliana and Nicolle). Know that I love you all—the end.

contents

introduction

When I decided to write a book about style, the first thing I wanted to do was make it real. No nonsense. No confusion. No talk about runway fashions that are unrealistic for the real woman. I wanted to offer the most useful advice on what to wear, so getting dressed would finally make sense. Well, here it is: real information, foolproof tips, and a closetful of secrets to help you discover style for yourself.

As you read this book, you'll identify your body type and the cuts and fits that flatter it. **You'll understand what clothing is right for you and what to avoid.** You'll learn about everything from the must-have basics that are the foundation for every great wardrobe to the accessories that provide a flawless finish. And, page after page, **you'll get the inside scoop** on the best tricks of the trade that have been well-kept secrets—until now.

Lots of books out there tell you what to wear, and magazine pages are filled with fashion dos and don'ts. But how many of them actually tell you *why* you should be wearing something, or what makes a don't a don't? *Real Style* gives you the answers to your style questions and explains the "why" behind it all.

Let me make it clear from the start that I don't presume to know everything about style. All my life, I've been learning through my experiences. When I was young, I spent a lot of time around designers because my mom was in the high-fashion business. I developed a fascination for clothing, and by the time I was twelve, I was making over everybody who'd stand still long enough.

When I got older, I worked as a personal shopper at Fred Segal, Hollywood's exclusive specialty store, where I helped women of all shapes and sizes—from celebrities to the girl next door—solve their issues about how to dress. I learned how to fool the eye with the right clothes, how to balance the most difficult proportions, and how to create a head-turning look on any budget.

My learning process has continued with my role on ABC's hit reality series *Extreme Makeover*, where I've worked with real women before and after their dramatic transformations. I've seen their confidence and self-esteem blossom right before my eyes as they realize the depth of potential that lives inside them. They simply needed help to bring it out.

Throughout my work, I've taken a long, hard look at what individual style is all about. Is it the clothes you wear—cut, fabric, proportions, and fit? Is it a knack for accessorizing—being able to toss a scarf around your neck or add a piece of jewelry that takes your outfit to new heights? Is it the way you shop—your talent for scoring a find in everything from high-end stores to thrift shops? Or is it how you feel in your clothes—a comfort level that shines through no matter what you're wearing?

Yes—it's all of the above.

Real style is about making choices that work for your figure and your personality. It's about creating your own successful look instead of following someone else's trend. It's about becoming a more discriminating shopper, so you stop filling your closet with the wrong clothes once and for all.

Most of all, it's about slipping into something and feeling good—in both body and mind.

My goal is to help make real style a part of your life. I want to open doors and windows and turn on the lights to let you see all the beauty you have—no matter how your body is shaped—and give you the confidence to go out there looking your best. I want to give you the tools you need to succeed, because in the end, *you* create your style.

The tips I'll share with you are proven solutions. Like your grandma's best recipe for chocolate cake, they guarantee consistent results— and they're even better when you put your own special spin on them.

To most of us, extraordinary style does not come naturally. Many of the "gorgeous" celebrities whose looks we would die for rely on the expertise of a skilled stylist—someone with a lot of fashion sense who can create the illusion of perfection even when it's not really there. Lucky them, huh? Well, lucky you, too, because now you have me.

Why do I know what looks good on people? Because, as I always say, "I see you, you don't see you." When you look in the mirror, your sense of perspective flies right out the window. Instead of seeing your entire body, you zero in on what you consider to be your flaws. If you think you have saddlebags, your eyes go straight to your thighs. If you think you have a bulging belly, you immediately stand sideways and check out your middle in profile. Sound familiar?

Starting now, those days are over. I'm going to help you recapture the big picture, so you can see your entire body in a clear new light. You'll learn how correct proportions and fit can create a balanced relationship among all the items you're wearing. You'll become your own cosmetic surgeon—trimming bulk here and adding contours there—except you'll do it all with the right clothing instead of going under the knife. So **get ready to take on your new image,** because you're about to learn some fashion facts that can change the way you look at style—and your body—forever.

Let's face it—no one is perfect. (Okay, some people are, but we won't go there, and yes, we're allowed to hate them.) It's just that the ones who look fantastic know how to hide their flaws and accentuate their best assets. They're real women with real bodies who work with what they have.

When you truly know your body and feel comfortable with it, you can look sensational all the time—attending a formal event or a business meeting, lunching with the girls, or just hanging out in your favorite jeans, T-shirt, and flip-flops.

In these days of makeover this and makeover that, we're all striving to change something to look just right. But you don't need to go to the extreme to get the incredible results you're looking for.

In *Real Style,* we'll go on a treasure hunt together. I'll be your guide, your personal shopper, your Hollywood stylist, and your best friend. And I promise to tell you the whole truth, page after page.

Some women were born with great style. And now no one will know that you weren't.

real
SAM SABOURA'S
style

CHAPTER 1

Getting to Know You

BODY TYPES

$\mathcal{H}$ow many times have you shopped for hours, only to end up frustrated and discouraged? You think that nothing out there is made for your body. Nothing looks good, no matter what the cut or shape. In fact, nothing fits properly at all. **Before you know it, a bad shopping day turns into a bad self-esteem day.**

You start believing that your hips are too big or your boobs are too small or your butt is too wide or your legs are too short. Your arms are too flabby or your shoulders are too sloped or your belly is too round or your waist is too long. You're convinced you'll have to go naked for the rest of your life—or at least go on a diet or go to the gym, because something just isn't right.

Wrong! You're just not shopping for the right body.

Until you identify your body type, you have no way of knowing what styles are best. To get on track, you have to figure out exactly what kind of body you have. When you do, you'll have a clear picture of what to wear for the way you're built and what to avoid at all costs. More important, you'll stop wasting money on clothes that still have the tags on and are too old to return. Reality check: These are not "inspiration pieces." They are just mistakes.

Before we go any further, I want to stress one important thing: No one—I repeat, no one—is one stock body type. Every person is completely unique and made up of a combination of many different types. So don't worry if you can't find your exact figure in the following list. Just select the basic shape that seems closest to yours, and use it as a general guide.

I also want you to keep in mind that your body is what it is. Sure, you can lose a few pounds or build some muscle or step up your aerobic exercise, but you can never transform the lush curves of an Oprah into the lean-limbed grace of an Audrey Hepburn. *And you don't have to.* When you realize this, shopping will be fun and enjoyable—the way it's supposed to be.

The Pear

Your figure is smaller on the top and wider on the bottom. Your shoulders are narrow, your breasts are small to average, your waist is slender, and your hips, thighs, and bottom are full. Your goal is to visually alter the proportional differences between your upper and your lower body to create a sense of balance.

Boatneck and off-the-shoulder tops are great choices to create a more pronounced horizontal shoulder line and balance the width of your hips. Avoid tight-fitting tops (I'm not talking about fitted here—I mean super-snug), which will exaggerate the difference between your top and bottom halves, and—you guessed it—make your hips and butt look huge. The same thing happens when you wear a belted dress or cinched waistline.

Pears should always wear dark colors on the bottom, taking advantage of the slimming effect of black, charcoal, navy, brown, and other deep tones. Low-rise pants work wonders to minimize your hips and help create a more balanced look. Straight-leg pants or ones with a slight flare do the same by adding width to the bottom of your leg, making your hips look smaller by comparison. A-line and circle skirts are perfect for you, because their shapes skim right over your trouble spots.

Stay away from pants with side pockets and pleats, because they just add extra bulk to your bottom half. By the same token, drawstring pants, with all that extra fabric gathered around your midsection, make your hips look big and broad. And we won't even talk about what they do to your butt!

Pants with a tapered leg are a don't unless you want to look like an ice-cream cone—and I'm guessing you don't. They make your legs look too skinny from the knee down and make your thighs and hips look wider. Please take a pass on this dated trend.

STYLE SOLUTIONS FOR THE PEAR

Best Feature: Upper Body

Your upper body should always be your focal point when you're planning an outfit. Since your goal is to minimize your lower half with simple, dark, solid bottoms, have some fun with your tops.

Look for brighter colors, proportional prints, and sexy necklines. Try a fitted top when you want to look curvy, and a looser, straighter style when you want some camouflage. Wear small shoulder pads—yes, shoulder pads—to broaden the top half of your silhouette and offset the fullness of your hips. Play with necklaces and earrings, because they'll draw attention upward. Also, consider your hairstyle in relation to your lower body. A fuller, sexier do just might give you some additional balance by adding volume to your upper half.

When choosing skirts and dresses, always try an A-line first. This style is a reliable classic, and it's tailor-made for your body.

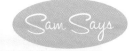

MIX AND MATCH

Mix-and-match separates are custom-made for the pear-shaped girl. No matter how big the difference between your top and bottom, you can buy exactly the size you need. You might also consider looking for tops one day and bottoms the next, making shopping a lot easier.

The Willow

You are tall and slender—the Nicole Kidman of your neighborhood. Your breasts are small, your waist and hips are narrow, and your legs and arms are long and lean. But what only you realize is that your willowy stature makes it difficult to find clothes that fit properly. If a size is small enough for your slim frame, odds are it will be too short in the legs and arms. On particularly bad shopping days, you have to sneak into the men's department just to find pants that are long enough.

Your goal is to make sure you wear clothing that is suited to your body type. You need pants and jackets that are long enough to cover your limbs, and you want to create proportions that keep you from looking too lanky. Your tops should always be a bit on the longer side, to balance the length of your legs.

When it comes to skirts, you shine in long ones, because your height allows you to wear them with grace. But stay away from the super-short mini. Though shorter skirts that reveal your slender legs are fine, a micro-mini will make you look like you're walking on stilts.

You can wear pants in just about any style—as long as they're long enough. They should be three-quarters of an inch above the heel in the back, with a break in the front and a hemline that covers the top of your shoe. Avoid buying a too-short pair just because you like them and they fit everywhere else. Unless there's enough fabric in the hem to lengthen them, they will never be more than well-fitting pants that are too short. Also beware of pants that have an extremely flared leg. They add too much weight to the bottom of your slender frame, throwing you visually off balance.

Though it's fine to flaunt your height with stilettos and the like, keep in mind that flats and lower heels are always a winner for the willow. They're chic and classic, and will keep you from towering over your shorter friends on days when you prefer to blend in.

In choosing outfits, try separates that cut your long frame in half. A flowy skirt with a high boot can bring interest to your lower body. For contrast, add a fitted tank or long-sleeved knit top. If you love wearing dresses, try belted styles that tie at the waist to play up your lean middle.

STYLE SOLUTIONS FOR THE WILLOW
Best Features: Height and Long Limbs

You're blessed with a willowy look—go ahead and flaunt it.

High-end designers cut and style their clothing with your body type in mind. Instead of searching for days to find three pairs of so-so pants that fit your budget, spend the sum total on one perfect pair that costs a bit more. You'll acquire a wardrobe of great-fitting clothing over time.

Go for contrast when you dress, layering to your heart's content. Your lean frame can handle the extra coverage, and you'll add style and dimension to your look. Try pleated skirts for fullness, textured fabrics for interest, and jackets and shirts with large collars and exaggerated cuffs. Wear lighter, softer colors. You have less to minimize, so darker shades can work against you by making you look too tall or too lean—and, yes, sometimes that is not a good thing. Also avoid super-snug clothing, because it can take you from slender to rail-like.

Sam Says

GO FOR PRINTS AND PATTERNS

As a willow, you're among the lucky few who can wear large prints, so wear them with wild abandon. They're striking, and you carry them well because they won't overwhelm your tall frame.

The Hourglass

You have a curvy figure, with a full bust, small waist, and full bottom. Some people accuse you of dressing too sexy when you're not even trying. You make a magnificent Marilyn Monroe at Halloween, and you have the most sought-after body in history. Embrace those curves! Women spend tens of thousands of dollars on cosmetic surgery trying to get a body like yours.

For starters, invest in a pencil skirt. It's sexy yet classy, and the slightly tapered bottom will show off your curvy figure. Team it up with a contrasting belt that defines your slender waistline and draws attention to it. Look for fitted tops that nip in at the waist and stop somewhere between the waist and hips, bringing the eye to one of your best features. Avoid full or blousy styles that can hide your body.

You have the option of going for a sexy look, like a low-rise pant with a flared bottom that will minimize your hip area and balance your hourglass curves. Play it up with a low V-neck or scoop top that reveals a hint of cleavage. Or you can take the more classic route with a higher-waisted pant or skirt that shows off your small waistline. Add a tank or spaghetti-strapped top that shows a little skin, or choose a long-sleeved fitted knit or body-defining T that's tucked in. You're one of the few body types who can pull this off, because of your minimal waist. The idea is to define your hourglass figure without getting carried away. Your curves should whisper, not shout.

Avoid cropped tops at all costs. They may show off your small waist, but they'll draw too much attention to your bust and make you look top-heavy. Also stay away from the opposite extreme: long, boxy tops. They disguise your curves and aren't even remotely flattering. The same goes for loose-fitting dresses that hide your narrow waist and make your body look shapeless. And to keep from looking like a double-wide, make sure your tops don't stop at the point where your hips are the fullest.

WRAP IT UP—I'LL TAKE IT!

A wrap dress is one of the most flattering styles an hourglass can wear. It's made to follow the lines of your body, showing a hint of cleavage, highlighting your waist, and baring your sexy legs.

Best Features: Curvy Body and Small Waist

Your natural curves give you built-in sex appeal. Your bust, waist, and legs are your best arsenal, so use them well.

Fitted clothing that hugs your curves will always be your best choice. You can be fitted and tasteful at the same time by wearing tops and dresses with a bias cut. They wrap and hug your best features, and fall a bit looser everywhere else. Stretchy fabrics are good, too, since they find your curves and show them off.

Wear shoes that are hot and sexy to showcase your legs. Add a fun belt or sash to play up and accentuate your small waist. Less is really more when it comes to prints and patterns, so it's best to wear solid colors on the top and bottom. Sometimes, just seeing the silhouette of your body is sexy enough. Bring in the prints with smaller, detailed accessories.

The Apple

You have a rounded figure, with a fuller bust and midsection, heavier arms, and shapely lower legs. You wonder why you never see your body type addressed in the fashion magazines. After all, the average American woman wears a size 14 or 16—depending on which survey you read—yet women in the media are usually no bigger than an 8. Now you can be as dazzling as the slinky girls, because plus-size fashion has evolved beyond the big-and-baggy look.

The key idea for the apple is to create lines where none exist. Since your body is round, drawing lines and angles on it with the right clothing will help to counteract it, creating the shape and curve you strive for.

Try a V-neck top with an empire waistline. The V will slim your bustline, the seaming under your breasts will provide lift and support, and the fabric below will fall loosely over your midsection for the perfect concealment. Fabrics that are more substantial are good, because they drape nicely over anything you want to hide. Tops with long sleeves are always a plus, but they should never cling to your fuller upper arms. Loose, flowy fabrics like silks, rayons, and gauzy cottons also make the grade. Wear a stretchy fitted tank or T-shirt underneath to add support, hide any bumps and bulges, and provide these lighter fabrics with a solid foundation.

Pants and skirts that fall in a straight line from the hip down and skim over your middle are smart choices. Keep in mind that anything that clings too tightly to the fuller parts of your body will put emphasis in the wrong places.

Prints and patterns can actually distract from the things you want to conceal, so they can be assets to the apple. Feel free to wear them with confidence, and break them up with a solid color here and there. A slightly larger print is best, particularly when the colors are low-contrast and the pattern is consistent. Smaller prints can make you look bigger, so stay away from them. Consider narrow vertical stripes, too, which create slimming lines on your body.

Stay away from pleated pants, pants with side or cargo pockets, or any style with detail or embellishment around your middle. This is not an area where you want to focus attention. Above all, don't wear tapered pants. They'll just make you look top-heavy and exaggerate your fuller figure.

The most important tip I can offer the apple is this: Don't hide your body where you don't have to. Every woman has some part of her that she's proud of, so find yours and flaunt it. Because you have the ability to look majestic, there's no need to take cover under oversized tops and dresses that drag you down. Besides being incredibly boring, these styles make you look bigger and unfinished, and you're way too fab for that!

STYLE SOLUTIONS FOR THE APPLE
Best Features: Fantastic Breasts and Shapely Lower Legs

I've never met an apple who doesn't have a gorgeous bustline, so don't be afraid to show a little cleavage when you're dressing up. And if you're one of the lucky ones who have great calves to match, kick up your heels and show your legs off for all they're worth!

Besides highlighting your legs by baring them from the knee down, your style objective is to wear clothing that offsets the roundness of your shape. Look for tops with a square or rectangular cut that stop just below the waist to counterbalance your fullness and conceal your tummy. Also try tops and skirts with asymmetrical hemlines. Their angular seaming and details intersect and cut the bodyline to flatter you from head to toe.

Clamdiggers are perfect for you, because they stop at the knee and bare the lower part of your leg. They're a great alternative to shorts for the summer months.

Separates are also a great way to break up your bodyline. For evening wear, a skirt-and-top combo may work better than a dress, because it's easier to find flattering individual pieces seemingly custom-fitted for your top and bottom halves.

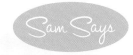

"X" MARKS THE SPOT

Wrap tops and halter dresses are perfect for the apple, because they create the line of the letter "X" across your middle. The X brings the eye into the centerline of your body, minimizing your torso with its diagonal lines and offering flattering camouflage.

The Rectangle

Feel boyish no matter what you wear? Do you get more compliments when you're in your boyfriend's or husband's clothes than when you're wearing your favorite dress? You're a rectangle, with shoulders, waist, and hips that are all about the same width.

You'll be amazed at how you can change the look of your body and create a more feminine image. Start by wearing belts. Skinny, wide, or in between, they're your best choice for accentuating—and creating—a waistline. Choose wrap tops and dresses that gather or tie at your waist, drawing diagonal lines that point right to it. Corset tops are also good, because they cinch in your middle and create the illusion of a curvier figure.

Drawstring pants are wonderful for you, because the gathering creates fullness in the hips to give the illusion of a waist. Don't wear extremely low-slung pants, because they'll make you look like a box. A slightly higher rise will give the illusion of the waist you're missing.

Boxy sleeveless tops are a no-no for you. They draw horizontal, masculine lines on your body, and you don't want more of those. Also avoid loose-fitting dresses. Their shapeless style will make you look . . . well . . . shapeless. And always make sure your jackets don't have wide lapels that add unnecessary width and square-ness to your upper body.

STYLE SOLUTIONS FOR THE RECTANGLE

Best Features: Arms and Legs

The key for the rectangle is to soften the lines of your body whenever you can. This means paying attention to fabrics and cuts and avoiding those that add unnecessary hard angles to your frame. Showing some skin is a good way to add softness, so choose sleeveless tops that are cut to bare more of your shoulder.

Team them with capris to bare some skin on the bottom, too.

Gauzy, flowing fabrics and silks and satins are always great choices. Curvy cuts, soft ruffles, and fluted edges all work overtime to balance your straighter lines. Show off your feminine side by wearing skirts and dresses, especially ones with asymmetrical hemlines.

When you are wearing masculine styles like blazers and trousers, add something feminine to soften the lines—a flower pin, a colorful high-heeled shoe, or a sexy lace camisole. Your waistline should be your focal point as often as possible, so your closet should be stocked with expressive belts, fitted tops and jackets, and skirts that have a higher waistline.

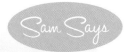

The Diamond

Your pear-shaped friends envy you for your slender bottom half, but they don't know the *other* half of it. You, too, struggle with balance— it's just upside-down—because you carry most of your weight on the upper half of your body.

The good news is, there are lots of ways to draw attention to your lower body and create the illusion of equal proportions. Think bright bottoms. Pants and skirts in vivid colors and prints will offset the size of your top half. Pleated and tiered skirts do the same thing by adding fullness to help balance your upper body. The flowing shape of palazzo pants is also a smart choice, because the wide legs run from hip to hem and fill out your lower half.

A short skirt is fine for the diamond, but keep the length within reason. A too-short skirt or dress will make your top half look larger compared with your slender legs, and the trade-off just isn't worth it.

Tops for the diamond are best in V-neck and scoop-neck styles that draw attention away from your broad shoulders. Avoiding boatnecks, horizontal stripes, or any kind of intense pattern on your top half will keep it looking leaner. These add unnecessary width to the shoulder line and draw attention to your larger torso. Epaulettes and shoulder pads are out for you, because they magnify your upper body.

STYLE SOLUTIONS FOR THE DIAMOND

Best Feature: Sensational Legs

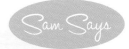

As a diamond, you should focus on the lower half of your body when getting dressed. Keep the top half simple and muted, and go to town on the low down.

Printed skirts and pants, shorter hemlines, and sexy shoes are everything you need to show off your legs. Minimize your shoulders and bust with deeper necklines, and camouflage the fullness of your arms with draped sleeves in any length.

Try a top that falls below your hips, creating the dropped-waist look without wearing a dress. Pair it with a tube skirt, which is shaped like a long tube and hugs the body, tapering slightly from the knee down and ending at the ankle. The coverage will fill out your bottom half while providing a lean, sexy look at the same time.

DROP IT!

If the diamond were stranded on a desert island with only one dress to wear, it would be one with a dropped waist. Reminiscent of the twenties and thirties, this is the classic flapper-style dress. The loose-fitting top hides your fuller upper body, bringing your great legs front and center.

The Half-Pint

You're actually in a class by yourself. You can have any of the body types addressed above, but the one characteristic that sets you apart is your short stature. You might have a stocky, athletic body, or you could be a petite version of the willow. No matter how you're built, one thing is certain: If you gain five pounds, it looks like ten.

To make up for your lack of height, you wear three-inch heels to the grocery store—just because. You struggle with the proper skirt length for your frame, and pants are always too long. Since it's not likely that you'll be having a leg-lengthening procedure in Switzerland anytime soon, you're anxious to find out what you can do to look longer and more proportional.

You can magically add inches to your height by wearing all one color. (This is called monochromatic dressing.) It makes your body look like one long, lean line, because there are no other colors to break it up.

Surprisingly, longer pant lengths will create height by visually elongating your leg, and are better still when paired with a medium heel. Keep pants simple and darker in color, with a flat front and a side or back zipper, because they provide an uncluttered line for your lower half. Choose a medium-low to a higher waist, since super-low-waisted pants will make your legs look shorter than they are.

When shopping for both tops and bottoms, look for seaming that adds vertical lines, which will make you appear taller. You're better off with patterns that are small and delicate—just like you—so avoid prints that overwhelm your short frame.

If you have longer hair, try wearing it in a cute, messy updo or a high ponytail that can work for day or night. Both will add some height to your frame. If you prefer a shorter hairstyle, that, too, can make you look taller because the length won't compete with your petite body.

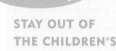

STAY OUT OF THE CHILDREN'S DEPARTMENT

Unless you're shopping for something simple like a T or tank, don't be tempted by the scaled-down sizes in the children's department. Most kids' clothes look like kids' clothes, and you're not fooling anyone but yourself.

Keep jewelry and purses simple and in proportion to the rest of your body. Choose small, delicate bracelets and necklaces. If you like long earrings, make sure the length is no more than one inch. Look for a scaled-down handbag, such as a clutch or pochette. The point is to complement your body, not make it disappear under piles of accessories.

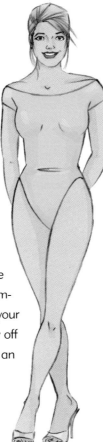

Best Feature: Your Petite Frame

For the half-pint, proportions are extra important. If an item of clothing is just a few inches too long or too short, it can make or break the big picture. You may want to put your tailor on retainer, because the subtle details—a nip here or a taper there—can help to finesse your overall style.

Keep things slim on your bottom half. A straight or boot-leg pant with a longer hemline will do wonders. When it comes to dresses and skirts, shorter styles work best as long as you've got the legs. If not, stick to styles that stop around the ankle, but no longer. Pair everything with some kind of heel to give you additional height.

On top, fitted works better. Solid colors rule most of the time, so when opting for a pattern or a print, keep it very simple. A vertical stripe works well, because it will help lengthen your torso. Just keep in mind that you don't have the size to carry off anything too big or bold. Add your own spin and interest to an outfit by finishing it with some funky accessories.

Foolproof Solutions to Common Concerns

There are many proportional issues that have been causing women angst since the fig leaf went out of style. But there are just as many solutions to correct them. When you follow the dos and don'ts for the body you're in, you'll start looking and feeling the way you've always wanted to.

Following are the most common concerns expressed by women about their bodies—and the best ways to correct them. This is the before-and-after magic of the right choices in clothing.

THE CONCERN	THE SOLUTION	THE WHY
Short neck	Wear V-neck and deep scoop-neck tops.	By showing more skin around your neck, you create the illusion of greater length.
	Try medium to long earrings.	The longer line of this accessory can visually lengthen your neck.
	If you have the face for it, cut your hair a bit shorter.	A cropped style will open up your neck and show it off.
	Avoid turtlenecks—mock or otherwise.	They make your head look like it's sitting right on your shoulders.
Long neck	Keep your hair on the longer side.	It will balance the length of your neck.
	Wear turtlenecks galore.	Covering up your neck with fabric will help avoid the swan look.
	Try shirts with higher collars, or turn up a traditional collar.	The height of the collar will cut the long line of your neck in half.
Broad shoulders	Wear V-neck tops.	The V draws attention down your body and away from your broad shoulders.
	Wear spaghetti straps and tank tops.	Straps cut the shoulder line in half. The broader the shoulder, the thicker the strap.
	If you're relatively slender, try a tube top.	It echoes the horizontal line of your shoulders to keep you in visual proportion.

THE CONCERN	THE SOLUTION	THE WHY
Broad shoulders (continued)	Wear tops with raglan sleeves, which have a diagonal shoulder seam.	Their slanted lines counteract your shoulders' strong horizontal lines.
	Wear dark-colored tops.	A dark color can minimize just about anything.
	Wear unstructured jackets and tops.	They soften your hard shoulder line with their relaxed look.
	Avoid jackets with lapels that point up to your shoulders.	This is the equivalent of drawing an arrow to your shoulders that says, "I'm a football player."
Narrow shoulders	Wear off-the-shoulder and boatneck tops.	The horizontal line adds width and focuses attention on your neck and shoulders.
	Wear shoulder pads. You can buy a pair that attach to your bra straps with Velcro.	Look for small ones that add subtle width to your upper frame.
	Wear sleeveless, boxy tops.	They create a broad, square shoulder line where you don't have one naturally.
	Wear horizontal stripes.	They visually broaden your shoulders.
	Have fun with epaulettes, ornamental shoulder tabs that you see on military uniforms or safari shirts.	They bring attention to the shoulder line, making it appear wider.
	Look for jackets with wide lapels.	They add volume to your frame, filling out your upper torso.
Flat chest	Wear tops with patterns, ruffles, cowl necks, or pockets over both breasts.	Embellishments play up your bustline by bringing attention to it.
	Wear tops with horizontal stripes.	Horizontal stripes make anything look larger, including breasts.
	Wear boatnecks and off-the-shoulder tops.	The wide necklines open the width across the collarbone.
	Work wonders with a halter.	It gives you a lift and pulls the breasts together for a sexy finish.
	Always wear a padded cup or push-up bra.	It can amplify your smaller bust and add the cleavage you're longing for.
	Wear fitted tops.	They will hug any existing curves and show them off.

THE CONCERN	THE SOLUTION	THE WHY
Full chest	Wear V-neck and scoop-neck tops.	These draw vertical or slanted lines down the center of your body, minimizing your bust.
	Wear wrap tops.	These create a cross-your-heart visual, distracting the eye from the heavy bust and making your waist look smaller in the process.
	Wear small collars and skinny lapels.	They draw attention away from your breasts.
Full arms	Wear tops with loose-fitting sleeves.	A loose-fitting long sleeve does the job well, and a three-quarter sleeve has the added advantage of baring the smallest part of your arm.
	Add a wrap if you must go sleeveless.	Cardigans, blazers, ponchos, and wraps are all stylish ways to cover your arms.
	Wear off-the-shoulder tops.	They play up your shoulders and neckline, while covering up and distracting from your fuller arms.
Short waist	Wear the same color on the top and bottom.	Monochromatic dressing gives the illusion of a longer torso by creating a clean, uninterrupted line along the length of your body.
	Wear narrow belts that are the same color as your top.	Matching belts to tops will visually lengthen your torso.
	Choose low-waisted pants.	The lower the waistline, the longer the torso appears.
	Wear tops with vertical stripes.	Vertical lines elongate the torso by forcing the eye to look up and down.
	Shop for tops in the petite department.	The proportions of petite tops are shorter, so you get a length that fits you properly.
Long waist	Wear high-waisted pants.	A higher rise elevates your waistline, shortening the length of your upper body.
	Wear pants without cuffs.	Cuffs shorten the length of your leg, making your waist look even longer.
	Wear wide belts that are the same color as your pants.	Matching belts to pants will add visual length to your legs by creating a continuous line of solid color.

THE CONCERN	THE SOLUTION	THE WHY
Long waist (continued)	Choose skirts and dresses that end just below the knee.	This length will make your legs look longer, balancing the length of your torso.
	Have fun with layered tops.	Adding visual interest with tops of varying lengths detracts from your long waist.
	Wear high-heeled shoes that are the same color as your pants.	The expanse of a single color will lengthen your legs.
Poochy belly	Wear a girdle.	It will hold the tummy in, smooth any rolls, and whittle a few inches off your waistline.
	Wear dresses and tops with empire waistlines.	The seam on an empire waist lifts the bust, which elongates the tummy. This style also provides superb coverage.
	Wear flat-front pants with a bit of stretch.	They create a clean, smooth line and offer the slimming effects and comfort of stretch.
	Shop for tops with ruching.	Gathers and pleating in the fabric along the seams hide problem areas in the tummy and waistline.
	Wear your tops long and untucked.	This eliminates the gathering around the belly that occurs when a shirt is tucked in. The top should be long enough to cover the pooch, and drape loosely to avoid any clinging.
Large bottom	Wear pants with a V-shaped yoke on the back.	The yoke sits just below the waistband on the back of a pair of jeans. It works to minimize your bottom, just like a V-neck does to minimize your top.
	Select pants that sit slightly lower on the hips.	The higher the waist, the bigger the butt looks.
	Always wear pants with back pockets. Keep their size in proportion to your bottom.	Pockets provide a visual distraction from the width of a larger bottom.
	Wear jackets with a defined waistline that are long enough to cover the hips.	You can create the look of an hourglass figure *and* cover up your problem spot.

THE CONCERN	THE SOLUTION	THE WHY
No bottom.	Fashion your own butt by wearing high-waisted pants.	They lift and separate the rear just like your best bra enhances your breasts.
	Wear pants that are fitted in the seat.	They give the illusion of a butt by hugging even the smallest curves.
	Try pants with smaller back pockets.	They will make your rear seem larger by comparison.
Big hips/thighs	Wear boot-cut pants.	The flare will put your lower body into proportion with your hips, making your thighs look slimmer in the process.
	Choose skirts with a slight A-line.	The shape of this skirt prevents the fabric from clinging to the parts that you're trying to conceal.
	Avoid shorts and skirts that stop at the fullest part of your thigh.	They can make your legs look heavier by emphasizing their broadest point with a horizontal line.
No hips	Wear wide belts and choose wide waistbands on pants and skirts.	Wide belts add visual width to slender hips, giving you volume where you need it.
	Choose pants with pockets.	These add size and fullness to the hips. Cargo pockets and elaborate pockets that sit higher on the leg and closer to the hip are best.
	Wear slightly tapered pants.	The slim lower leg plays up your hips and makes them appear wider.
Thick ankles	Wear longer, flared pants.	This tip works like an A-line skirt for your ankles. You get coverage and no cling.
	Wear sling-back shoes.	They make the front of your foot look longer, minimizing the fullness of your ankle. The back strap rides low, so it will not call attention to your ankle's widest part.
	Look for dark-colored boots that hug the ankle tightly with elastic panels.	Any bunching around your ankles will add to their bulk. A tight, streamlined boot will make ankles look slimmer, just like a corset.

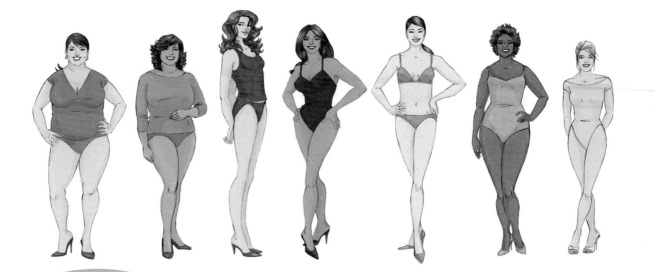

WARNING This book is not called *The Constitution of Style*. Amendments are always allowed, and there are exceptions to every rule. If you can pull off a look that's on your don't list—fantastic. This means you're learning to see what looks right on your body no matter what the experts say. And that, girls, is what real style is all about—knowing what works best for you.

CHAPTER 2

Of Epic Proportions

THE PROPER FIT

When you see someone walking down the street who appears to have perfect style . . . when a friend always seems to look "just right" . . . , chances are she is dressed in proper proportion for her body.

Most bodies—even the "perfect" ones—are not perfectly proportioned. In fact, many of us have one leg that is slightly longer than the other, and top and bottom halves that are at opposite ends of the spectrum—never mind all the stuff that lies in between. Proportion is all about the relationship of size and shape between one thing and another, causing the overall look to be either pleasing to the eye or out of balance. **Finding pieces that visually adjust the proportions of your body will bring your clothing and your body into perfect harmony.**

Dressing in proportion means that you see your clothing as a corrective tool. Every item of clothing has the potential to alter the proportions of your body, celebrate your greatest assests, and minimize even the most stubborn flaws. And you can do it all by choosing the right clothes, with the right fit, right now.

Choosing Your Battles—Shirts and Tops

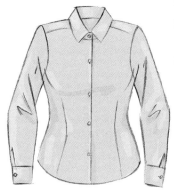

When you try on a top and it fits just right, all of the elements come together and the planets seem to align. You know it's a keeper and worth every penny. But do you have any idea what makes this one so much better than the other twelve tops you tried on that same day? You're about to find out.

Something as simple as a well-fitting T-shirt or tank top, a basic knit, or the right button-down shirt may be all you need to change the way your body is perceived by others—and even by you when you look in the mirror. Clearly, the magic starts with the right fit, but things really heat up when you figure out exactly what your body needs—the details that bring your body into flattering proportion.

For example, the collars, straps, and necklines of your shirts, tanks, and tops play a huge role in adjusting the proportions of your shoulders and bust visually. If your top balances the relationship between the two, no one will ever know you've struggled with a flat chest for years or inherited your father's broad shoulders.

The type of sleeve you choose, right down to the size of the cuff on your favorite button-down shirt, can make a world of difference. Consider the stopping point of your sleeves—whether long, short, or three-quarter. The amount of skin you elect to show and the style of cuff you decide upon will determine how long or short your arms appear to be.

When it comes to the width and length of the tops and Ts you wear, you can balance the proportions of your body simply by choosing a style that contrasts its shape. A rounder torso is balanced by a straighter, boxier cut. A more square-shaped trunk needs softer lines, tighter fits, and angles to create curves and movement. The same goes for long and short waists—choosing a top that is the opposite length of your torso can help fool the eye into seeing the harmony that's not there naturally.

So the motto is this: Choose your battles when you choose your tops, and the proportional issues you've been struggling with will be replaced by the spoils of victory—and a well-balanced top half, too.

THE RIGHT FIT FOR SHIRTS AND TOPS

Collar A shirt collar should button to fit—even if you're never going to button it—with no more than one-quarter inch of space between your neck and the shirt, allowing enough room for comfort. Consider the width of your shoulders in relation to the size of your collar. Broad shoulders need large collars; narrow shoulders need small ones.

Shoulder The shoulder seam on any shirt should stop at the end of your shoulder—not past it, not before it. If the seam is too high up on your shoulder, the top will look skimpy and shrunken. If the seam drops off your shoulder, the look is baggy and sloppy.

Bust If a T-shirt or top pulls across the bust or the placket gaps open when you button it, it's too small. If the shirt has darts or seams on the sides of the chest or underneath it, make sure your bust fits comfortably within them.

Sleeve The sleeve should fit cleanly without too much extra fabric, which can add weight. Some women like to show the entire wrist, revealing a delicate, feminine body part. Others prefer to wear a sleeve that ends just at the top of the hand. Both lengths are acceptable.

Cuff When the cuff on a long-sleeved shirt is buttoned, it should hit just above or below the wrist bone, depending on your personal preference.

Width If there are more than two inches of extra fabric on either side of your body, the top is too big. If you absolutely love it and it fits well everywhere else, find a good tailor who can take in the sides or add darts to reduce the width.

Length As a rule, an untucked shirt should stop no lower than the end of the rise of your pants, or at the bottom of your zipper. But always consider the length of your torso in relation to your tops. Shirts that are too long can make you look short, and shirts that are too short can throw you out of proportion.

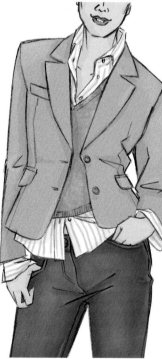

FITTED, GIRLY JACKET

Perfectly Proportional Jackets—the Long and Short of It

The right jacket or coat can be fitted or boxy, long or short, or somewhere in between. In all cases, it is a beneficial tool for correcting proportion. Besides completing the look of just about any outfit, it can fool the eye into seeing a well-balanced body no matter how you're built—as long as you choose the correct style for your body type.

SHORT JACKETS

A fitted, girly jacket is in a class by itself—a wardrobe essential whose elements are female all the way. With lean lines through the torso, waist, and arms, it is tapered and darted for shape with princess seams. The collar and cuffs can be exaggerated or scaled down, with design details like larger buttons or piping that add a more feminine touch.

A girly jacket usually stops at the waist or just over the hip. By defining the waist and flattering the hips, it balances the pear's torso by filling it out, creates a waistline for rectangles and apples, and is made to measure for the half-pint's shorter frame. The willow can wear a cropped, fitted jacket well, because it accentuates longer legs with distinction. In most cases, the diamond should avoid this style, because it may add unnecessary bulk to a fuller torso.

A girly jacket can also have a boxy cut and stop at the waist or just above it, which brings to mind the fashions of Coco Chanel. Perhaps you've heard of her? She was a famous French couturière in the early 1920s whose empowering, sophisticated clothing designs liberated women from the corseted styles of the early part of the century. Her chic renditions of women's jackets have become timeless classics, favored by fashion icons like Jackie Kennedy Onassis.

Though boxy, this jacket is utterly ladylike. It works well for slender women with a smaller bust, and can cut the length of a long torso. It balances curves by contrasting them with straight lines, it's nicely unexpected with jeans, and it adds structure and width to women who have narrow shoulders. Best of all, it's been knocked off about a thousand different times at every price point.

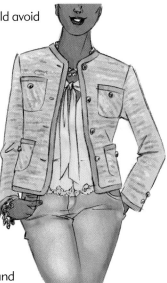

BOXY, GIRLY JACKET

LONG JACKETS

A longer jacket or coat can be anywhere from three-quarter-length, extending to the hips or mid-thigh, like a pea coat . . . to the knee, like a trench . . . or all the way to the ankle, like a maxi. It can be double-breasted, nipped in at the waist, and even belted, incorporating design details that aid in correcting every proportional issue. Your height will play a major role in determining which longer styles are right for you. (Basically, the taller you are, the longer the coat you can wear.) So, naturally, the willow has free rein in the long-jacket division.

The pea coat is perfect for the pear, because it's essentially the A-line of jackets. It adds volume to the upper body, stopping just over the hips and thighs and minimizing them as a result. It is great for the diamond because it resembles a drop-waisted dress, playing up the legs. And it's

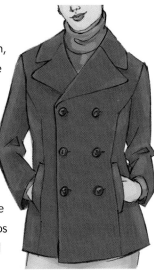

PEA COAT

LOOKING LONG AND LEAN

A jacket that is cut higher under the arms will elongate your torso, because the seam that runs along the side of the jacket starts higher and creates a longer vertical line down your body. It also makes your arms appear longer and more slender—a two-for-one deal!

The first time you try on a jacket like this, it may feel a bit strange and maybe even a little snug. But as long as the jacket is comfortable in the shoulders and bust—and you don't feel as if you're wearing a straitjacket—you'll get used to the difference and love what you see in the mirror.

WHITTLING A WAIST

Rectangular girls and no-waisters, take notice! A peplum jacket—which is short, with a fitted waist and a flare or flounce that falls just beneath the waist—will give you the streamlined waist you've always wanted. Wear it with everything from skirts to pants to your favorite jeans.

just right for the half-pint, who dreams of wearing a longer jacket that won't overwhelm her frame—though she'll always want to add a heel for extra measure.

The rectangle and hourglass will love the waist-defining benefits of the belted trench coat or knee-length jackets that are tapered slightly at the waist. The apple and willow will fall for the coverage and length-defying quality of the maxi coat.

Once you've determined the jacket style that's best suited to you, you need to be sure that it fits properly. The following guidelines explain how each component of a jacket should come together for maximum impact.

TRENCH

Collar Can be small, large, or nonexistent—depending on the size of your shoulders, bust, and torso. Keep the size of your collar in harmony with the size of your body.

Shoulder Can be padded or soft—depending on your shoulder line. The seam should stop at the end of your shoulders.

Arm Higher armholes will lengthen your torso. Lower armholes are less structured, and will accommodate larger arms. Leaner sleeves work for slender arms, wider sleeves for fuller ones. Long arms can have a cuff at the wrist to break up the long line. Shorter arms should stay with clean, simple, and uninterrupted sleeves to add length. Sleeves can stop before, at, or below the wrist, depending on your preference and arm length.

Chest It should zip or button to fit, even if you never intend to close the jacket. Darts are a plus to define a small bust and accommodate a fuller one. Button size and placket details should balance the size of your torso, small or large. When closed, the jacket should allow freedom of arm movement without pulling the jacket up or opening across the chest.

Bodice If the style is relaxed or boxy, no more than two or three inches of extra fabric should be present on either side of your body. If the jacket or coat is fitted, it should hug the curve of your body without grabbing or showing flaws.

Length A jacket can stop at the waist, hip, mid-thigh, knee, mid-calf, or ankle. The style of jacket, your height, and any areas you want to conceal will guide you to the perfect length.

Skirt Shapes and Lengths

When choosing a skirt, you should consider two important components: shape and length.

A pencil skirt is a flattering style when you need to add definition to your lower half. It has a distinctive curve in the hip, and a pronounced taper that ends at the hemline and accentuates your curves. It can sit higher, at the smallest part of your waist, or can be worn low on your hips, and it works for both long and short waists. Every body type can wear a pencil skirt—as long as your legs, from the knee down, are ready for a close-up. It looks best when it's a bit fitted to hug the body, and the correct length is at the knee or just above it. For ease of movement, many pencil skirts feature a slit or kick pleat in the back.

The mermaid skirt is a variation of the pencil style, with fluting on the bottom. It should be worn a little longer, stopping just below the knee.

Gorgeous on every frame, an A-line skirt is slim at the waist and graduates to a fuller bottom. This style can be worn higher on the waist, or can be slung lower on the hips to create a casual, beachy look. The ideal lengths for an A-line are at the knee and just below it.

A-LINE

PENCIL

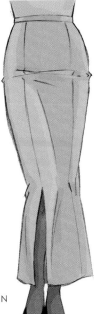

COLUMN

A long, columnlike skirt adds drama to a tall or leggy frame by lengthening the bodyline. It provides excellent coverage, and can hide big ankles and calves with ease. A long skirt should stop at the ankle or just below it. Taller apples and diamonds of any height will enjoy the uninterrupted line of a longer skirt that balances the upper body. Rectangles, pears, and half-pints should approach this style with caution.

A tube skirt is a longer version of the pencil skirt, and is good for the hourglass, diamond, and half-pint. Usually made of a stretchy material, it contours the line of the lower body in its entirety, hugging its shape and stopping at the ankle.

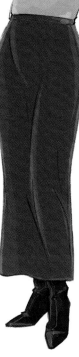

TUBE

real style secret

HIDING FLAWS ON THE BIAS

Bias cut means that the fabric of a garment is cut on an angle, across the grain. The fabric wraps around you like a spiral, hugging your curves and falling loosely in other areas, effectively hiding places you might not want to show. A bias-cut garment will look small when you see it on a hanger, because it collapses in on itself when it's not being worn.

Don't be afraid to try one on, because it's a terrific way to create camouflage. It's not for everyone, and you'll know immediately if it works for you because you'll be able to see which parts of your body it hugs and where it relaxes. Also keep in mind that the seams on a bias-cut dress or skirt will not always lie flat. This is normal—like wrinkles in linen—and the benefits of fit far outweigh the subtle lumps of puckered seams.

Any body type with standout legs can flaunt 'em with a mini. It should sit on the hip and stop above the knee—anywhere but at the widest part of your thigh. A micro-mini is very revealing, baring the uppermost part of the thigh. Besides requiring killer legs, this style screams youth. Even if you're an athletic forty-year-old with lean, rock-hard limbs, reserve the micro-mini for the twenty-somethings and under, please!

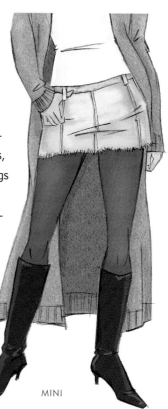

MINI

An asymmetrical skirt has an uneven hemline that can be longer on one side than the other or feature different lengths all around. It draws angles on the body, creating lines and curves where none exist. It also lets you show some leg without going overboard, and can camouflage a variety of lower-body issues, such as heavy thighs, imperfect knees, and fuller ankles—depending on the length you choose.

The asymmetrical skirt should not be too tight, since you want to draw the eye to the unique hemline, not to any body bulges. This style works best when the varying lengths are not too different from one another, because extremely short and long lengths are tricky to wear.

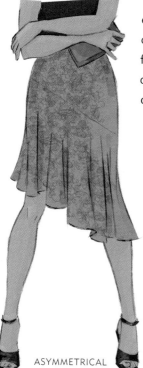

ASYMMETRICAL

Waist A high-waisted skirt should hit the top of the waist, mid-waisted should fall at the center of the waist, and low-slung should sit just atop the hips. The waistband of the skirt should fit comfortably, with no extra fabric, gapping, or pinching.

Hips Depending on the style, skirts should hug the hips or skim very close to them. Fuller skirts or novelty styles may flare from the top of the hips outward.

Thighs For curve, your skirt should hug the thigh area slightly, tapering its way down. For camouflage, it should flare from the top of the thigh to the knee and beyond.

Length Skirts can stop at mid-thigh, the knee, mid-calf, the ankle, and the floor. The style you choose depends on your height, legs, and areas of concern.

real style secret

THE TOWEL-AND-MIRROR TRICK

Your best skirt length is generally determined by the shape of your legs. To help figure out where your skirts look their finest, here's a useful tip that was taught to me by one of my best friends:

Holding a towel lengthwise in front of you at your waist, stand in front of a mirror. (Obviously, you need to be bare-legged to do this.) Move the towel up and down until you find a length that flatters your legs. This easy exercise will cut your next shopping trip in half, because you'll already know what skirt lengths to look for.

A few basic rules are:

- A short skirt should fall at the leanest part of your thigh.
- A mid-length should fall either above the knee or below it at the narrowest part of your upper calf.
- If you have thick legs or ankles, it's all about long skirts.

The Pant Conundrum

Choosing the right pant can completely change the proportions of your body, balancing the relationship between your top and bottom halves. To do so, you'll have to consider your lower body in three parts.

THE RISE

I usually recommend a low-rise pant, because it works best for most body types. Please keep in mind that when I say low-rise I mean just a bit below the belly button. So don't be intimidated by this popular style and assume it's only for younger girls. In fact, don't knock it until you've tried it, because you may be very pleasantly surprised.

Low-rise pants correct proportions by minimizing fuller hips and thighs, lengthening a short-waisted woman's upper body, and making everyone's butt look smaller. So, if you're dealing with any of these issues, low-rise pants are a win-win-win solution.

High-rise pants can visually shorten a long torso and create a butt where genetics failed you. If you're short, they can elongate your legs. And last but not least, the higher the rise, the more coverage for the belly area, flattening your tummy like a girdle.

HIPS, BUTT, AND THIGHS

When it comes to flattering your hips, the style of pant you choose hinges on the shape of your lower body. Smooth, flat-front pants create a clean line and get a sweeping "yes" across the board for nearly all body types.

Pleats are dated and should be laid to rest. They were invented to provide extra comfort and movement in the hip and thigh area, but they do little for correcting proportions and end up looking sloppy. If you have no hips and want to create the illusion of fullness, you're better off choosing pants with interesting pocket treatments, which are a more modern alternative to pleats.

real style secret

INSTANT TUMMY TUCKS

High-rise pants hold the tummy in like your best girdle—a wonderful trick of the trade.

Pants with a side or back zipper, a flat front, and no pockets can make you look five pounds thinner. Add a sleek, thigh-length undergarment, and you'll be amazed at the change in your silhouette.

LEANER LEGS WITHOUT EXERCISE

Ironing a crease into a pair of pants or jeans is like drawing a vertical line on your legs—slimmer in a flash! Try a heavily pressed crease down the front of the pant leg, just like on a man's dress trousers. The line draws attention to the center of the leg, luring the eye away from the hips. Who would have thought that your iron could make you appear slimmer?

GORGEOUS GLUTES ON DEMAND

When you really need an extra kick in the rear, look for an undergarment with fanny pads. They are surprisingly comfortable, easy to wear, and excellent for special-occasion dressing. This is one of Hollywood's best-kept secrets for filling out and lifting your backside.

Pockets have a major impact on side-to-side body proportions. Very few women would opt to add bulk to the hips, thighs, and butt even if they're in gym-toned shape. It's the lack of side pockets that keeps the lines of a body uncluttered, bulk-free, and more appealing. If you prefer pockets, try one of these four flattering styles: side pockets, which run vertically along the seam and are almost invisible; slash pockets, which run on a diagonal across the hips; coin pockets, which are only about three inches across and sit just under the waistband; or the classic scoop pocket, which is usually found on a pair of jeans.

And then there's the butt. In my opinion, a good butt is one that attracts attention without bowling people over. The shape of your butt should define your backside without throwing you off balance. Design details on your butt can make or break your body proportion. If you have a larger butt, look for details that aren't too big or too small. Huge, flapped pockets will make your butt look larger, as will tiny, delicate ornamentation. Moderation is key.

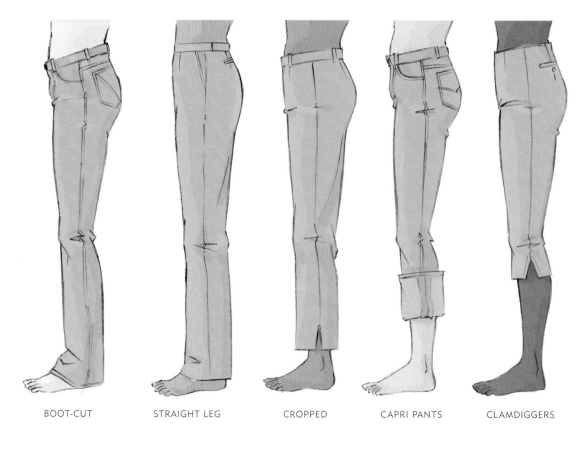

BOOT-CUT   STRAIGHT LEG   CROPPED   CAPRI PANTS   CLAMDIGGERS

If you have a smaller butt, you can add some dimension by wearing pants with no back pockets. Higher rises and tighter fits also accentuate the curve. If you have no butt at all, look for details galore to call attention to it. Three-dimensional back pockets (like the raised pockets with a fold in the middle that you see on the back of cargo pants) or flap pockets will add substance, and those with ornamentation and stitching will create the illusion of a well-rounded backside.

LENGTH AND LEG STYLE

One of the best ways to add length to a shorter leg is by wearing your pants a tad longer. If you toss a same-colored higher-heeled shoe into the mix, your legs look longer still. And if the hem of your pants covers the shoe completely—without falling into a sloppy pool at your ankle—you've got legs for days.

You can play down the length of long legs by wearing shorter hemlines, since showing a bit of skin on the bottom of the leg makes it appear shorter. Choices include cropped pants, which stop at the ankle; capris, which hit the top of the shins; and clamdiggers, which stop at the knee or just below it.

When you're trying to offset fuller thighs, hips, and torso, you just can't beat the benefits of a boot-cut pant. Think of the way an hourglass figure is shaped. Its perfection lies in the balance—fuller on top and fuller on the bottom, with a hot little waistline in the middle. Enough said.

The cut of a straight-leg pant gives you a beautiful smooth line from the bottom of the hip all the way to the bottom of the leg. Because this leaves no stopping point for the eye, all that's apparent is length and balance.

Now that you know what style is best for you, use the following guidelines to ensure that your pants always fit you like a glove.

Waist The waist should button to fit comfortably without pulling or stressing the closure. Whether the pants sit high, medium, or low on the waist, there should be no gap at the sides or the back. The waistband should not dig into your tummy when you sit or bend over.

Rise The rise of a pant resembles a U. It starts at the top of the fly and runs around the underside of your body, connecting at the seams of the crotch and continuing up the center seam of your rear, stopping just below the waistband at the back of the pant. When you're standing, the rise should lie flat and smooth. When you sit, it's okay if it bulges a bit. The rise should hug the contours between your legs without riding up, and there should be no extra fabric that droops below the end of the zipper.

Hips The pant should fit easily over the curve of the hip, without pulling the fly apart or causing any bunching or creasing. If the pant has front pockets, they should lie flat and go undetected. If you can see the outline of the inside pockets through the fabric of the pants, the hips are too tight.

Butt The backside of the pant should smoothly hug the curve of your seat, with no bunching or tight creasing where the end of your cheek meets the back of your thigh. There should be no extra fabric on either side of the back center seam, unless the pant has a loose fit.

Thighs If the pant has a boot cut, it's okay for the thigh area to be fitted to show off the flare of the leg and the curve of the hip. But if you can see any bumps, bulges, or cottage cheese, the fit is too tight. If the leg is straight, the fabric should merely skim the thighs. For a palazzo leg, it should not touch the thigh at all.

Leg The fit of the leg from the knee down depends on the style of the pant. It can be straight, full, flared, tapered, or cropped.

Length Ideally, your hem should be three-quarters of an inch shorter than the bottom of the heel of your shoe. If you're not wearing shoes—and you always should be when considering your pant length—the hem should stop at the floor below the end of your bare heel.

The Impact of the Right Dress

Shopping for a dress can present a significant challenge. Your entire body comes into play—not just your hips or your waist or your breasts—so you have to be focused on every detail to find a garment that accentuates your strong points, corrects your proportions, and makes you look brilliant. The good news is that there are many styles to choose from, and they're all available in a variety of fabrics for every season of the year.

Having entered the fashion scene in the fifties, the A-line dress has endured for half a century—and it's no wonder. This style is fitted at the waist and flares out like the letter "A" toward the hem, and is complimentary to every body type. An A-line can be worn in all lengths, but shorter pear-shaped women should keep it at the knee or just below, showing some leg to balance the slight upper body. The top of the dress can run the gamut of style, so give your upper body what it's asking for—halter, plunge, strapless, tank, or spaghetti strap.

The empire dress, inspired by the Elizabethan era, is fitted on the top and open just above the chest, with a scooped or square neckline. A seam runs horizontally under the bust, and the dress either flows down loosely from that point or is fitted in the bodice. It's well suited to a smaller bust, because the snug breast area brings attention where you need it. What's more, the empire waist camouflages the belly and lengthens short waistlines.

When buying an empire dress, make sure it is well tailored. If not, you may be mistaken for being pregnant, and that is not a good look unless, of course, you actually *are* expecting a child. Apples and women with larger busts can wear this style as long as the neckline is cut lower and the breast fits neatly without spilling underneath the seaming.

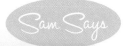

Sam Says

LEARN TO ACCEPT THE SHIFT AND PULL

There's a little dance that every woman does when she wears a strapless dress. To keep her dress—and her bosom—in place, she yanks up the top of the dress and moves it from side to side, a move known as the "shift and pull." In many cases, this little ritual is performed subconsciously. It's a natural consequence of donning a strapless dress, and probably can't be avoided.

Q I'm a larger woman who's going to a formal high-school reunion, and all my friends will be wearing strapless dresses. How can I fit in without showing a lot of skin?

A It's true that a strapless dress will play up fuller arms, broad shoulders, and a larger bust. But if you have your heart set on wearing one, there is a solution. A strapless dress can be paired beautifully with a dressy cardigan or wrap. You'll still get the elegant, formal look, but the parts you want to play down will be covered up nicely.

A strapless dress can be sexy, sophisticated, or sporty, putting your neck, shoulders, and arms in the spotlight. This style works well if your shoulders are broad, because it creates a horizontal line across the bust that balances their width. If your shoulders are small or sloped, it will only drag them down farther. A strapless dress shines in any length, offering versatility to make it work for most body types.

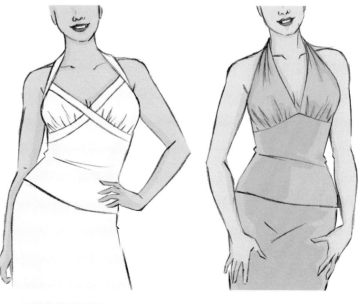

X-FRONT HALTER   PLUNGE HALTER

A halter dress has a sleeveless bodice that wraps or ties around the back of the neck and is often backless. It comes in A-line, pencil bottom, long, and short, so you're sure to find one that works for your body type.

Everyone looks good in this style, as long as you have the arms to show off—or a wrap for coverage. The variations on the upper half of this dress are endless, accommodating the proportions of any body. Halters can be X-front or plunging, bringing interest to the center of the torso and minimizing the bust. They can also wrap across the bust, creating a keyhole and a small peek of cleavage.

Smaller busts gain cleavage from a halter because of the lift and pull around the back of the neck, and are further flattered by cowls, which drape loosely in a swag from shoulder to shoulder at the neckline; ruffles that are fluted along the neckline; and minimal halter styles, which hug the front of the neck and cover the upper chest to expose sexy shoulders.

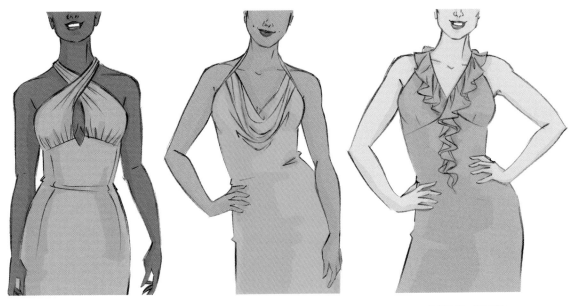

KEYHOLE HALTER   COWL HALTER   RUFFLED HALTER

THE HITCH WITH KNITS

Knit dresses, though gorgeous to look at on the runway and in fashion magazines, are difficult to wear in real life. As a stylist, I always hesitate to pull a knit dress for a client, because it's like putting a piece of gauze over a grapefruit. You can still see the grapefruit in all its bumpy glory through the gauze; imagine what it does to a real woman. Select this risky dress with care, and take a friend along before you buy it, for an honest second opinion.

THE HIT OF SLITS

Slits were invented to give women who have less on top something to show off on the bottom. They are especially good to showcase the great legs of apples and diamonds. Slits can be in the front, back, or on the side of your favorite dress, all producing good results. And the bonus? Ease of movement!

Halters can hide the bulge between the side of a large breast and a fuller arm. They also cut broad shoulders with an angular line, and can play up narrow shoulders by making them the focal point of the upper body.

A wrap dress features a bodice that is cross-wrapped by fabric. It can have either a high or a low neckline, and can be haltered, sleeveless, or sleeved. A phenomenon of the seventies, it was brought into vogue by Diane von Furstenberg (Google her, ladies—knowledge is power). This dress affords both comfort and style, because it can be adjusted to grow and shrink with you. It remains a staple today because of its many body-balancing benefits.

The wrap dress offers versatility that compliments several body types. It can either wrap around the body and tie at the side of the waist, or it can simply zip up the back or side, with the "wrap" style already sewn into the dress. The crisscross effect of a wrap dress gives you a touch of cleavage and defines your waist.

It is excellent for the apple, because it accommodates bust, belly, and all. It's a waist-defining "must" for the rectangle and hourglass, and a great choice for the willow and half-pint. But it's a "no go" for the diamond and the pear, because extreme variations between the top and bottom halves throw this style off course.

The shift is the *Breakfast at Tiffany's* little black dress. Sleeveless—yet offering lots of body coverage—it features a horizontal neckline that grazes the collarbone or extends to a boatneck. It maximizes your bust, shows off toned biceps and triceps, and emphasizes the shoulders. Though not the curviest of dresses, it usually adds some shape with darts and seams in the bodice. The bottom of the dress can be slightly tapered toward the hem like a pencil, or straight toward the hem like a column.

The spaghetti-strap dress is one of the most popular styles, and the easiest to wear for most body types. It can be cut straight across the chest or have a sweetheart neckline that dips slightly in the center to show off a little cleavage. The options for the bottom half are endless, ranging from a narrow sheath to a full skirt. Think of it as a strapless dress with support, which makes it good for fuller-chested women. Also, the skinny straps cut the shoulder line—ideal for broad shoulders.

A dress with sleeves provides the coverage you need to hide both heavy arms and skinny ones. But this is a tricky point, because, though instinct tells us that women should wear sleeved dresses to cover up trouble spots, I have yet to find one that doesn't make fuller arms look like sausages. The only remedy is a loose sleeve, which can risk delving into mother-of-the-bride territory. So here it is, plain and simple: If you find one that flatters you, buy it. Otherwise, we defer to the willow and her lean-limbed sisters, who can almost always make this tough style look beautiful.

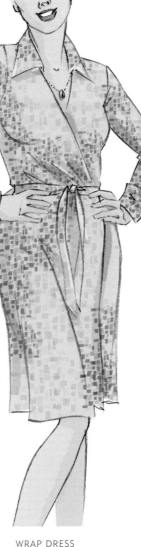

WRAP DRESS

You'll know you found the perfect dress when every part of your body feels good in it. The following guidelines will show you how to achieve that feeling.

THE RIGHT FIT FOR DRESSES

Arms Whether a dress is long-sleeved or sleeveless, the armholes should be cut low enough to accommodate the arms and the sides of the breast without grabbing, spilling, or showing the side of your bra. You should be able to raise your arms comfortably without lifting the dress.

Chest The breast should fit easily into the neckline of the dress without flattening. If the dress has darts or cups for support, the chest should sit within them without spilling above or below. There should be no pulling across the chest or creasing beneath it, and there should be enough room to accommodate some sort of bra should you choose to wear one.

Back The back of the dress should have a smooth fit without showing any rolls, bumps, or bulges, and there should never be any extra flab hanging over the seams. If there is a zipper in the back of the dress, it should zip easily without puckering and allow for freedom of movement.

Rib cage The rib cage, from below the bust to the top of the waist, should be fitted but still comfortable. A tighter bodice will help correct your posture, making the dress look that much better.

Waist The waist is where the bodice ends and the skirt of the dress begins. It is the most important part of the proportions of a dress, and should appear to be the smallest part of your trunk. The waist should be as fitted as possible along the sides to enhance your curves without causing a crease at the tummy. In a dropped waist, the fitted area runs all the way down to the upper hip. If you have a round tummy, the dress should have design details—like ruching or gathers—around the waist to conceal any belly bulge.

Butt In a fitted dress, the fabric should slightly hug your backside and cup its curves. In a full, loose, or straight-skirted dress, your butt is not the center of attention, so the fabric should fall loosely over it in a flattering line.

Hips A loose dress or one with a fuller skirt should skim the hips and flare slightly below them. A fitted dress will hug the hips, enhancing your contours without stressing the fabric or causing a crease. Make sure you can sit or bend comfortably at the hips.

Thighs A dress should be smooth along the thighs, and never be so tight that the thighs are smashed together to the point where you can't walk naturally. The dress should conceal any bumps, bulges, or cottage cheese in the thigh area, and the seams should always lie flat—unless the dress is cut on the bias.

Legs The dress should always bare the most flattering part of the leg.

Length The style of dress will determine the right length: mid-thigh, knee, mid-calf, ankle, or floor. When in doubt, ask your tailor to help you find the perfect length.

CHAPTER 3

The Building Blocks

MUST-HAVE BASICS

Real style begins to emerge when you have a strong foundational wardrobe that you can build on to create outfit after outfit. Without these basics, your closet can be filled with clothing—yet you still have nothing to wear. Trust me, I've been there. On the flipside is a wardrobe so simple, plain, and unimaginative that nobody notices you when you walk into a room. I've been there, too. Having the right fundamental items in your wardrobe means being ready for anything and everything.

Basics are meant to be grab-and-go pieces that you can always wear with confidence. Some will be relatively inexpensive and can be easily replaced, like T-shirts and undergarments. Others will cost a bit more, such as a designer handbag or a cashmere sweater. Whatever the case, they always work, and they are the heart and soul of your best and most stylish looks. The point is to create a foundation of clothing that can adapt to all sorts of social and professional situations. And even if you wear them a few times in the same week, no one will ever notice.

Basic Colors

The building blocks of your wardrobe should be made up of basic colors that offer flexibility, allowing you to mix and match them with everything you own without trying too hard. Of course, it's perfectly fine to have staples that fall outside these color guidelines, adding personality in a rainbow of complementary hues. But, to get started, you should focus on the essential colors. The following chart defines them and explains how they work as components of your basic wardrobe.

COLOR	THE "WHY"	BEST FABRICS	CHOOSE FOR
Black	The mother of all basic colors, it's slimming and sleek, and can look dramatic or conservative—and everything in between.	Wool, cotton, cashmere, silk, satin, rayon, and blends	A classic pantsuit or skirt, a little black dress, a sexy fitted top, basic heels, pumps, flats, a clutch bag
Navy	It's classic, sporty, and a good darker color for daytime.	Nylon, wool, cotton, and poly blends	An office pant or skirt, blazer, sporty outerwear, a pea coat NOTE: *Don't try to match navy to navy, because it will never work. Instead, wear it with a contrasting color*
Gray	It's businesslike, muted, a little masculine, and sometimes serious.	Wool, cotton, jersey, and cashmere	A business suit, dress, cozy sweater, winter accessories like scarves and hats, workout gear such as T-shirts and sweats
White	It's fresh, clean, and summery—your best choice for a crisp look when it's hot. And nothing is better for breaking up patterns.	Lightweight cotton	A fitted button-down shirt, a layering tank or T, summery pants, shorts, capris, sundresses
Brown	It's rich, sophisticated, and expensive-looking. It serves as a good alternative to black, and looks best in the fall.	Leather, wool, silk, or cotton	A leather jacket, a high-heeled boot, a classic loafer, an evening top, a fall dress for daytime, a tweed pant
Camel	It's casual yet elegant—a great neutral that complements the warm colors in your closet and goes great with jeans.	Fine-gauge wool, cashmere, cotton, and leather	A lightweight turtleneck, a daytime moleskin pant, a corduroy blazer, a work trouser, a trench or raincoat, daytime leather basics like shoes, bags, and belts
Khaki	It's easy, preppy, conservative, and says approachability.	Cottons and other casual fabrics	A chino pant, a fitted cotton jacket, a sporty pencil skirt, shorts, capris

The Little Black Dress

The little black dress—the LBD—is a wardrobe essential that can take you from work to dinner, from a wedding to a funeral. It has its place in fashion history, and will continue to be a basic item of the best-dressed woman. There is no more classic or versatile addition to a wardrobe, and if you buy correctly, it should last for years.

It's best to have at least three versions of the LBD: one for warmer weather, one for cooler weather, and one that is dressy enough for evening. This is a garment that should endure beyond just a few seasons, so it's important to focus on fit and proportion and to avoid styles that are "all the rage." You never want your little black dress to be too trendy.

The fabric should be a durable cotton or wool, capable of holding up to several cleanings without fading or pilling. The look should be clean and simple. To make it work for day or night, simplicity and staying power are key.

real style secret

THE LBPT

Who says the little black number has to be a dress? Meet my new variation, the LBPT. The "little black pant and top" can serve the same purpose as its more famous counterpart, and still make you feel comfortable on any occasion. So invest in an exceptional pair of black pants, and team them with a special black top to suit the event.

The Universal Black Pant and Skirt

The perfect black pant and skirt are probably the most fundamental items a woman can have in her wardrobe. As staples, they should be updated as needed on a seasonal basis, so you always have them for both warmer and cooler months. When purchasing something as basic as a black pant or skirt, don't be afraid to spend a bit more money. A good designer brand that has worked for you in the past is best.

The basic black pant should be lightweight wool or cotton, and should be versatile enough to take you to work or out to play. Wool, in particular, is very durable and lasting, and is available in a tropical weight suitable for summer wear.

Make sure the pant is tailored for your body type, with seam allowances that can be let out or taken in as you grow or shrink. In this way your investment is protected, and you can get away with gaining or losing a few pounds without having to buy another pair.

When shopping for a basic black skirt, look for a pencil style or an A-line. This basic should never be longer than just below the knee. The perfect skirt is classic at the office, and elegant with a heel or boot for a night out.

The idea here is to cover a lot of ground with one skirt and one pair of pants. So don't select detailed, memorable pieces, because you won't be able to wear them as often.

Basic Jeans

Denim has always been a basic, because of its ease of wear and durability. You should have at least two pairs in your closet: a medium wash for everyday, and a darker pair that can be a versatile substitute to dress up your days and nights. Medium-wash jeans are the balance in color between light and dark denim, and look best with lighter shades on top. When you opt for tops in black, brown, and brighter colors, switch to a dark jean.

Dark denim has the ability to be dressed up and worn at night, and is a "must-have." I am constantly amazed at how it saves the day when I need to be well dressed for a dinner or event but wearing dress pants is not on the agenda. These days it is acceptable in a variety of situations, so treat it like a great black pant. You'll end up looking chic *and* feeling comfortable.

Knit Tops

Knits are wonderful basics that are a notch above your everyday cotton shirts and Ts. Wool, cashmere, and fine-gauge cotton are the best options, since these natural fibers are easy to care for, they breathe, and they last.

Wool is one of the most widely used fibers in a knit. If you find it to be itchy, you can combat the issue by wearing a camisole or a body-hugging T underneath it. Merino wool is a finer gauge of wool that tends to be less irritating. But if it still itches, switch to a soft cotton, or splurge on cashmere. Though cashmere *is* wool, it is a fine and rare form of it that feels incredibly cozy. There's no denying that cashmere is one of the most luxurious fabrics in the world, and it can last a lifetime when cared for properly. It is available in many different price ranges, and you should buy only what you can afford.

Q I love cashmere sweaters, but they're generally so expensive. I've started seeing inexpensive ones at my local department store. What's the difference?

A Cashmere comes from the undercoat of the long-haired Kashmir goat, which lives in the colder climates of the Far East. Its quality varies from silky to coarse, from single-ply to double or more, which explains the difference in price. Also, the inexpensive "cashmere" that's popping up around town may not be cashmere at all, but merely better sheep's wool touted as cashmere. Check labels carefully before you buy.

Truly deluxe cashmere has a denser weight and thickness, which translates to a higher price tag. But it's a sound investment, so save your money, shop around, and capture your cashmere off-season, when it's on sale.

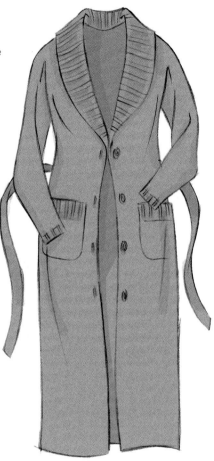

ROBE-STYLE KNIT

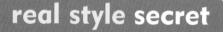

real style secret

CASHMERE CARE

Because cashmere is expensive and delicate, we immediately think that we must have it dry-cleaned. Wrong. Dry cleaning can make your cashmere rough and ruin its soft touch. The best way to care for your cashmere sweaters is by hand-washing them in a gentle detergent made especially for knits and delicates, or a mild soap that is used to launder baby clothes. Then place them on a towel, work them back into shape, and dry them flat.

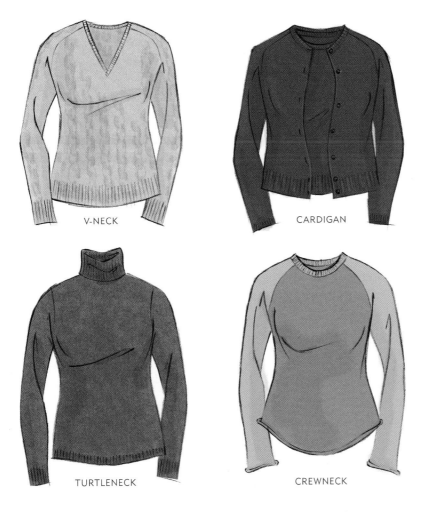

V-NECK

CARDIGAN

TURTLENECK

CREWNECK

Cotton is my old standby when it comes to a knit, since it can be worn year-round. Comfortable, affordable, and tasteful, it rarely pulls or pills, making it a good alternative to wool and cashmere.

Try it in a crewneck or V-neck sweater, which looks fabulous when layered over a crisp white shirt. Let the shirt hem show a bit, pull out the collar, flip over the cuffs, and push up the sleeves for a fantastic, preppy combo. Choose basic colors first, then throw a few more into play for some fun.

Cardigans come in a variety of styles—from button-downs to zip-fronts to hoodies—and you should own at least three or four. Wear one over a dress, as an alternative to a blazer at work, or as a substitute for a jacket at night. Knit hoodies are casual, and are best when fitted. Make sure you have one in basic black to toss on over anything, but also have fun with bold colors.

A turtleneck is a sleek choice if you have the neck to carry it. I suggest having at least two in your closet for the cooler months. It's terrific in a cropped style with a wide waistband teamed with jeans and boots in the fall, and looks stunning with a denim jacket or a long trench or pea coat. Try one in camel, chocolate, or a soft pink.

A robe-style knit makes a great classic—belted or wrapped, hip-length or longer. I suggest buying one on the thinner side to avoid bulking you up, and in a rich, dark color like brick red, black, or brown. It's wonderful as a layering piece, or as an alternative to a long jacket.

Shirts and Blouses

Your foundational shirts and blouses should be a bit interesting, so they can do the job of changing your look and expressing your personality. You should always have more tops than bottoms, because tops are more memorable and you can't get away with wearing them as often.

A white cotton button-down shirt is a "must" in long and short sleeves. Capable of looking both professional and casual, it has incredible versatility that will get you out of a bind when you have nothing else to wear.

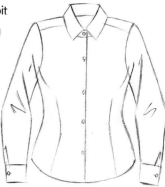

WHITE COTTON BUTTON-DOWN

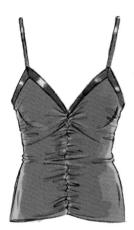

SEXY BLACK TOP

A sexy black top is the basic you can always throw on and feel good in without giving it much thought. It can be a woven blouse or a knit, but it must stand alone as special and different from the rest of your basics. Have at least two or three for variety.

A printed top in any style is a surefire way to break up the same-old same-old. If you are on the wild side, show it off with an animal print or a vivid pattern. If you are more conserva-tive, try a stripe or a floral for a clean, sweet look. Printed tops layer well under a jacket or sweater, and let you have some fun within the world of basics.

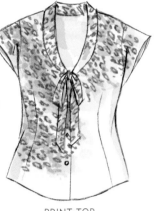

PRINT TOP

Casual shirts in bright colors and patterns are an important component of your basics wardrobe. These include polos and other styles that are just a tad dressier than your favorite Ts. Find ones that flatter your body type, and wear them when you want to feel slightly more put together.

T-Shirts and Tanks

There really is no end to your need for basic Ts and tanks. Feel free to own as many as you want, as long as you have a handful that fit you like a dream, can be worn somewhere besides the couch, and are in colors that look good on you.

Crewnecks, V-necks, and scoop-necks are easy layering pieces, cute with a blazer and jeans, and the quintessential no-brainer. You can get variety not only with colors, but also with sleeve lengths, fabrics, and styles.

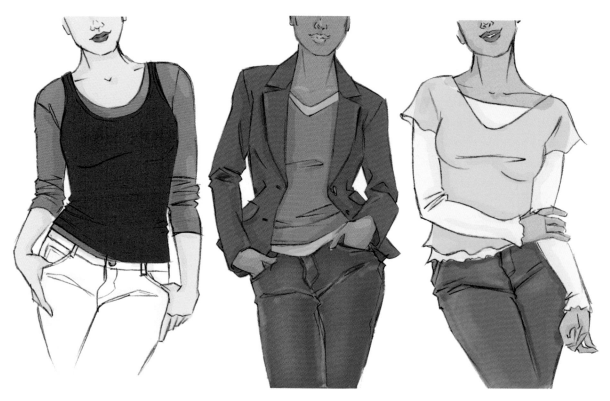

LAYERING Ts

LAYERING TANKS AND Ts

T-shirts and tank tops take on a vibrant and colorful dimension when you layer them. This is one of the easiest and most inexpensive ways to get a new look out of your existing wardrobe and make your basics work overtime. Choose two tank tops of the same cut and style in coordinating bright colors —like purple and turquoise—and layer one over the other. Or layer a short-sleeved T over a long-sleeved one. You can even try a tank over a T-shirt or under a scoop-neck T for a fashionable finish.

It's smart to have at least five each of long- and short-sleeved Ts in different colors. Because they're relatively inexpensive, T-shirts are the most renewable items in your basics closet. So don't be fooled into thinking that no one can see the stains or small holes that seem magically to appear, especially in your favorite white Ts. Replace them as needed to keep them fresh.

A tank top should be as comfortable as your favorite T. If you have broad shoulders, a thicker strap will offset them. If you have narrow shoulders, you should look for thin straps that won't compete with your slight shoulder line. Smaller busts should wear a tank with a built-in bra to maximize, but beware of the "shelf bra" that may flatten the chest. Fuller busts should choose styles with a slight V or sweetheart neckline in a thicker, stretchy material for support. When you find the style you love, buy it in basic colors like black, white, gray, and chocolate, and then add some bright, fun hues for variety and spice.

Jackets and Outerwear

Nothing completes and polishes a look better than outerwear. As the final layer of your outfit, it should be considered even before your jewelry and accessories. A jacket should be an effortless basic, and you should have at least two of the following styles.

A girly jacket in a fitted, cropped style can be worn with jeans, dressier pants, and skirts. Look for one in a texture or subtle pattern, such as tweed, corduroy, or velvet.

A denim jacket is one of the most fundamental and versatile pieces of outerwear you can own, and is perfect over everything from casual pants to dressy dresses. There are plenty of styles made just for women, and they tend to be more fitted, with feminine details, so they don't look like you raided your best guy's closet.

A blazer is an enduring classic, offering you a hundred and one looks. It's best to have two of these in your closet—one dark, one light. This is truly the "everything" jacket, so make sure it fits well and is in proportion to your body. A blazer is the one item that can correct just about all upper-body flaws, especially with shoulders and waistline, so have it tailored to fit.

A trench coat, pea coat, and three-quarter jacket all work as basics. It's essential to have a longer, dark colored jacket to wear at night—something simple enough to wear over everything from jeans to an evening dress.

Footwear Basics

Your basic shoes should be simple and functional. This is not the time to play Carrie Bradshaw à la Sex *and the City* by stocking your closet full of once-in-a-lifetime footwear. That little treat comes after the basics are in place. This is the time for common sense, comfort, and style, and your must-haves include heels, flats,

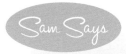

Sam Says

AVOID DENIM WITH DENIM

In spite of a denim jacket's incredible versatility, you don't want to wear it with a pair of jeans or a denim skirt. If you do, you may look like you're wearing a leisure suit, so opt for the contrast you get when you pair denim with other colors and fabrics.

boots, sneakers, and sandals. Buy what you love, and always remember that comfort and style go hand in hand. Don't sacrifice one for the other.

Your shoes can be the focus of your entire outfit. You can almost always tell a woman's personality and character by the shoes she is wearing—and people tend to check them out first—so make sure yours are worthy of the attention.

Most of the time, the more money you spend on a shoe, the better the quality. And since your whole body rests on them as your sole means of support and balance, they are just as important as a good bed.

Black, brown, nude, and camel are the most common colors for basic shoes, because they work with almost everything in your wardrobe. Once you have a few pairs in these colors, you can branch out and add different shades and styles.

Your basics should include a few high-heeled shoes, with an open toe for the warmer months and some pumps for year-round. Open-toed shoes work only if you have good toes—and you definitely know whether or not you do. At all costs, avoid toe cleavage—bunched-up toes that don't fit well into the open point of a shoe.

Look for heels that can go comfortably from day to night, affording a traditional look for the office and capable of dressing up a pair of pants or jeans for the evening.

The heel should be thin and graceful. Chunky heels are made for young girls who need more balance because they are not comfortable walking in heels. If you think a thinner heel is not comfortable, I challenge you to do some research. You'll be surprised at how things have changed. Women who absolutely can't wear a high heel should opt for a kitten heel, which is still delicate and slender but only an inch or two high.

Flats are essential for casual days, and can also serve as dressy shoes for a special lunch or afternoon event. Having a flat in basic black is best, and from there you can expand your collection. You have a lot of options to choose from, because flats currently feature as much style and design as the hottest high heels on the market. Choose a round-toed ballet flat or a sexy, pointy toe.

A boot brings out the savvy city girl in anyone. One pair in a basic color like black or chocolate will do for starters. They'll make you look taller when worn with a mini, they're super-fashionable with jeans, and they do a bang-up job of disguising fuller calves and ankles. Just remember that even though boots are on your basics list, they stay on reserve for the cooler months of fall and winter.

Sneakers can be functional or fashionable—or both. They're kicky with cargoes and other casual pants, and you can find them in a huge variety of styles. Some are simple and classic white; others are way out there, with architectural design elements, bright colors, and reflective everything. The sky's the limit here.

Sandals are the first footwear in history—timeless classics that should always be included in your spring and summer basics. A good pair of black or brown leather sandals is a smart investment, because they'll coordinate with most of the

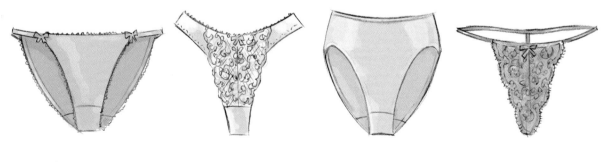

STRING BIKINI   THONG   HIPSTER BRIEF   G-STRING

colors in your wardrobe. You can add fun and personality with inexpensive and disposable versions, like flip-flops. They're easy to wear, and they go with everything under the sun.

Undergarments

This is where it begins for every woman every day. A good undergarment means a good foundation. In the old days, women didn't dress for their bodies, they dressed for their undergarments, and there is a huge difference between the two. I am a firm believer in this concept, and will explain it in more detail when I talk about evening and event dressing. For now, let's review the undergarments you should always have on hand.

Basic panties should be bought in nude, white, and black. The fun colors and sexy styles can get filtered in later. Always choose seamless ones, which really do eliminate panty lines. They're made in a slick, smooth material, with narrow elastic that is wrapped in the same fabric. You can find them in a variety of styles—bikini, thong, brief, G-string, low-rider, boy short, and tap pant—so pick the ones that are most comfortable for you and suit your outfit's needs.

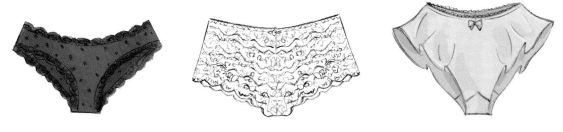

LOW-RIDER   BOY SHORT   TAP PANT

Q What is the fashion rule regarding bra straps showing under tank tops? Is this okay, or just plain unacceptable?

A This is a tricky one. My immediate response is to say no—it's not okay. But, truth be told, it's a difficult look to avoid. I would much rather have you show a bit of bra strap than go commando with no bra at all. So here is my solution. Whenever possible, try to match the color of the bra to the tank, so if it shows, it looks intentional. If you can't, try a nude bra with a very skinny strap, so it doesn't compete. You can also look for a bra that comes with clear latex straps. At least everyone will know you're trying to be discreet. One final word: When you're dressed for a special event, visible bra straps are completely unacceptable.

Look for bras in nude, white, and black in seamless styles, too, to maintain the no-show look. Basics can include soft cup (comfortable support with no underwire), underwire (strips of flat wire under the cups for added support), T-shirt (smooth, seamless, and molded), demi (an open, low-cut neckline that reveals more of the upper breast), and racerback (cut higher on the shoulders with a T-shaped back).

Certain clothing styles demand a special bra. Depending on the cut of the dress or top, you may have to add a strapless, demi, plunging, push-up, or

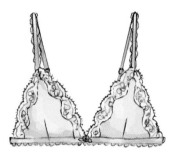

SOFT CUP

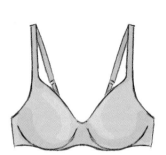

T-SHIRT BRA

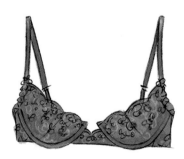

DEMI-CUP

padded version to your basic bra wardrobe. You can meet a lot of these needs by investing in a convertible bra, which can be worn any number of ways. I admit such bras can be like a puzzle sometimes, but they really do the trick. Having one on hand in nude and another in black can save the day.

Camisoles have multiple uses, and are a must under sheer tops. Nude, white, and black are essentials, but colors like blush pink or baby blue are also good to have. Wear a fitted one under a dressy top, an itchy sweater, or a suit. Select one in a fuller cut to wear under a blouse, either open or closed.

A camisole should be able to stand alone as a top, so don't buy it if it's strictly underwear. Ideally, it should fall into that blurred line between lingerie and tank top. Look for fabrics that are not too delicate. (Lacy camisoles are both feminine and basic.) Your favorites will get plenty of wear, so make sure they are easy to care for and can be thrown in the wash.

Hosiery, in my opinion, is becoming passé. I realize this statement may create some controversy and ruffle a few feathers, but I still stand by it. Other than a beautiful sheer nude or black, I say forget it. (And don't wear "suntan" pantyhose —ever.) Opaque, patterned, and textured tights are fine for the fall and winter, and work especially well with boots and a miniskirt.

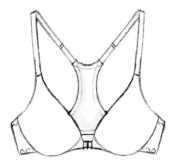

RACERBACK

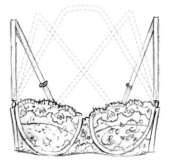

CONVERTIBLE

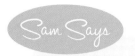

Basic Foundation Garments

Foundation garments are one of my favorite topics because they offer a helping hand when you need one. No one has a perfect body—and if you do, we don't want to hear about it. Besides, even the most glorious of us could use a bit of help here and there.

Today's options focus on comfort, and resemble well-engineered works of art. These are not your mother's girdles. The latest trends in foundation garments place as much emphasis on style as on function, making them the perfect basics. In fact, undergarments have become so popular and accessible that they are no longer tucked away in the back corner of your local department store. Endless variations of slimmers and body shapers abound, filling the racks and walls of the lingerie section.

For some women, wearing a slimmer is an everyday affair. For others, the purchase hinges on a specific occasion. Either way, you'll have to examine and identify problem areas to determine where you need help. The good news is you have lots of choices.

Tummy-control panties give you mild support and come in several torso lengths, ranging from just over the belly to right under the bust. Choose the amount of coverage and control you need.

The mid-thigh slimmer is styled like a bicycle short, and slims down the tummy, waist, hips, and thighs. A girdle-style slimmer gives you maximum control, with stronger Lycra and targeted stitch-

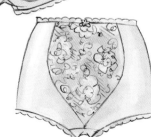

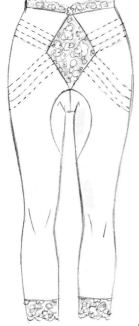

THE GREAT DISAPPEARING ACT

I still can't figure out why some women insist on wearing white underwear with white shirts and pants. White under white looks . . . uh . . . white! Your best choice is a seamless bra or panty in nude. I promise you—like magic, it will disappear into thin air as soon as you put on your clothes.

ing to trap and reduce your areas of concern. A pantyhose style is also available, and both are the ideal solution under dresses that show off the curve of your lower body. I don't recommend either of them under pants unless they're specifically designed not to show a line at mid-thigh.

A mid-calf slimmer is your best choice when your hemline drops lower or when you're wearing pants. You can find it in both a girdle and pantyhose style, ending just at the calf and giving your legs an all-over slimming effect.

When shapers and undergarments do their job, you can wear your regular size in clothing and feel more confident. Some will do it so well that they'll take you down a whole size. Yes, this is reason for celebration! Make sure that when you need an undergarment for a special occasion, you buy it before you purchase the outfit—just in case you do drop a size.

Now you have it—everything you need for a solid wardrobe foundation. These building blocks will get you off to a great start.

CHAPTER 4

Forever in Blue Jeans

DENIM

Denim has been around for hundreds of years, and it's no wonder. Jeans are the most durable and versatile clothing you can own, and they're incredibly easy to wear. **Sliding into a pair of jeans is the best thing you can do when you want to feel like "you."** Your favorites become a second skin—they know your every curve, and they mold to you over time to become individually yours. Denim has become such a fashion staple that you see it everywhere—from the raw styles on the street to the most exclusive runways and designer collections in the world.

Today, it is totally acceptable to wear denim with just about anything to just about any event. Jeans are rugged. Casual. Comfortable. And yes, ladies, they're also sophisticated and sexy. By the time you get to the end of this chapter, you'll be amazed at the kind of mileage you can get out of these fashion basics.

Haven't had the pleasure of an exceptional pair of jeans yet? You have no idea what you're missing. Finding them may not be the easiest thing on earth, but it can be the best thing you ever do for your wardrobe.

I have been acquiring multiples of my favorite jeans for the last year. I have them in a smaller size for when I want to feel sexy and cute, a larger size for when I just want to be "comfortable Sam," and one size in between for when I don't want to think at all. I have some jeans that I toss in the dryer, and some that I don't. I have some in a darker wash and some a bit lighter, though I'm the only one who can tell the difference.

Jeans come in so many shapes, styles, and washes that you could shop till you drop. And you may have to! Before you get excited about all the possibilities, keep in mind that jeans can be very hit-or-miss.

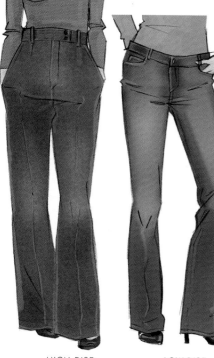

My guess is that you're already familiar with this problem. I'm sure every one of you has at least a few pairs of jeans currently collecting dust in the nether regions of your closet or drawer. Shopping for them can be a real project, and all the variations can make it even more difficult. So let me share a few facts that will alleviate some of the stress over buying jeans.

Low-Rise vs. High-Rise

Are you a low-waisted or high-waisted jeans girl? Well, unless you have absolutely no butt or are dedicated to the fashions of the last century, you should be a low-waisted fan.

I'm not saying that high-waisted jeans are completely passé—far from it. Jeans with a high waistline can create a curvy bottom if you don't have one, and can make your legs look longer if you're short. They are a fun throwback to the sixties and seventies, and can work wonders to hide a belly. But that's about all. If you want to make a statement that looks very current, find yourself a pair of jeans with a low waist. I promise you you'll love the body benefits.

HIGH-RISE　　　　　LOW-RISE

Low-waisted jeans are flattering to almost all figures. So get over trying to pull them up past your belly button, and let go of the idea that they are just for your daughter and her girlfriends. Once you get used to having your jeans ride a bit lower, you'll never go back to the high and dry.

Stretch Jeans

Stretch jeans are available with two-way stretch, the most common, which will "give" either up and down or side to side, depending on how the fabric is cut. (Try pulling on the fabric to see which way it moves.) You can also find four-way stretch that gives in all directions. Either way, stretch jeans are super-comfortable, because they move with your body. They also do wonders for holding it all in and effectively eliminating the gap syndrome at the back of the waist. Always try stretch jeans a size smaller, since they usually "grow" after a few wearings.

Washes

Denim comes in a variety of washes, and my personal favorite is a darker one. It's more flattering, gives you a wider range of tops to work with, and tends to look more expensive. Dark denim is appropriate around the clock, and, like your favorite basic black pant, it has a slimming effect. The deep blue color makes it virtually a neutral, so it matches just about anything.

Medium washes are more casual. Look for vintage pairs that have truly been around for a while, or for ones that have been put through the "aging process" to lighten areas like the thighs and butt. Both are already broken in for you, and have a wonderful, velvety soft quality that you can't find in a new pair of jeans. Just be prepared to spend a little more.

Lighter denim is reminiscent of the frosty days of the eighties. If you have an ancient, well-loved pair that have been weathered to the color of a pale winter sky, wear them at home on cozy nights in front of the fire. Preferably alone.

Jeans can come in a number of different fades and treatments that give them

Sam Says

HERE'S WHY
LOW-RISE JEANS
ARE ON THE RISE

- They minimize the curve of larger hips and thighs, making them a sure bet for the pear.
- They are the ideal camouflage for a short waist because they lengthen the torso.
- They prevent that scrunched-in-the-middle look that the apple can get from high-rise jeans with a defined waist.
- A medium-low-rise jean can help hold in a big bottom without any spillage.

real style secret

character and a more worn-in feel. Some look like real wear and fading. Others are more trendy and feature light-colored streaks all the way down the leg. Some come tattered and ripped, and others have paint splattered on them or are overdyed to appear "dirty." No matter what you're looking for, you can probably find it—and you'll wind up paying a pretty penny for design elements that may be yesterday's news by tomorrow.

In my opinion, most of these over-the-top styles are too contrived. They may be fine when tossed into the novelty-jean category to break up your basics, but let's be honest: Jeans don't naturally fade in such extreme patterns, so whenever I see this style I think they're trying too hard to be vintage. You're better off investing the time and money to find a real pair of vintage jeans at a good thrift store.

"Whiskers" give you the look of jeans that have aged naturally. They appear in stripes across your lap and behind your knees—places where jeans fade naturally on their own just from the movement of your body. They can look very unrealistic on the rack, because you don't see the design detail come to life until you actually put the jeans on. So give them a try for a cool and vintage look.

Novelty Jeans and Denim Skirts

The term *novelty* refers to jeans that have some action, some detail, some bells and whistles that make them different from your basics. Maybe they have a wider waistband; slash pockets and a finished hem, like a man's dress pant; or embroidery on the back pockets or down the leg. Whatever doodad they feature, they can add some fun to your denim collection. But open up your pocketbooks, girls, because they're going to cost you.

Denim skirts fall into the novelty-jeans category because they are a variation on a theme. All the rules of denim and a well-fitting skirt apply here. Choose one in a shorter style, because that's what works best for most body types.

Denim skirts are cute and fun when the summer heat prevents you from wearing your favorite pair of jeans, and they are brilliant in the fall with a knit, tights, a blazer, and a pair of boots. They can look fresh without much effort, and I highly recommend having one in your denim mix.

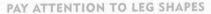

PAY ATTENTION TO LEG SHAPES

The cut of the leg can dramatically affect the way your jeans fit. If you want to look your best in a pair of jeans, follow these simple guidelines:

The boot-cut jean is incredibly popular these days, because it flatters so many body types. Keep in mind that we're not talking about the elephant bells that some of you may have worn in the late sixties. The twenty-first-century version of a boot-cut is barely flared at all. It's almost straight, with a slightly wider kick at the bottom that usually starts just below the knee.

A straight-legged jean is one that is the same width from the knee to the ankle. To determine if a pair of jeans fits this category, simply fold the leg in half to see if the cuff lines up width-wise with the knee.

This style suits short women, because the straight line makes your legs appear longer. It's the solution for apples, rectangles, and long-waisted women, too, because it creates a straight, lean line from the waist down.

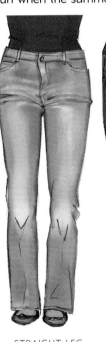

STRAIGHT LEG   BOOT-CUT

The Proper Fit

Your jeans should be your trophies. It may be a challenge to find them, but you'll eventually land the pair with the right fit. And when you do, it's a good idea to buy that style in multiples—even in different washes.

To ensure a well-fitting jean, look for these elements. If any part of you is spilling over the waistband, set vanity aside and go up one size. If doing so gives you a gap in the back of the waist, see your tailor, who can easily alter it for a nominal fee. This gap is common, and does not mean that the jeans don't fit. (It happens because every woman's waist differs in relation to her hip size, and it's impossible for manufacturers to design a jean to accommodate every body type.) Belts can help, but sometimes they make the problem worse by cinching in your waist.

The rise is the area below the waistband that runs from the top of the zipper to the joining seams at the crotch. Your jeans should hug this area comfortably, without being too tight or "grabby," and there should not be any extra length below the end of the zipper. Otherwise, you'll end up looking like you are wearing men's jeans with a long, sloppy line in the crotch area.

It's okay for a pair of jeans to be a bit tighter when you first buy them or when you pull them out of the dryer. Denim has a tendency to stretch, so your jeans will feel looser after about a half-hour of wear. Keep in mind that hips and thighs are the first places where jeans stretch out, so don't get them too loose in these areas. Always look for comfort, and avoid bagginess.

To get a proper fit in the butt, you'll need a good friend or an honest salesperson who is not going to tell you that your rear looks perky just to make the sale. Failing that, a small compact mirror will do, so you can check out what's happening behind you.

The seam should not ride up your butt. Contrary to the opinion of some, this does not make your bottom look better. Nor should the rear be too roomy, since it will make your butt look droopy. Jeans will "give" in the butt as you wear them throughout the day, so keep this in mind when shopping. You want to find a happy medium.

real style secret

THE RIGHT LENGTH

The ideal length of your jeans is three-quarters of an inch above the bottom of the heel of your shoe. Just to be safe, always buy them at least a quarter-inch to a half-inch longer, because you won't know the final length until after they're washed. So never do any alterations without laundering them and tossing them in the dryer first—or air-drying them, if that's what you plan to do over their lifespan.

If you need to shorten them, make sure you get a tailor to do the job so you can have the "original hem" put back on. No matter how many times you wash your jeans, you can never get the hem to look the same as the factory did. However, a good tailor can remove the hem, shorten the jeans, and reattach it without detection. This is the only way to alter jeans properly. Simply putting in a new hem and stitching it with orange thread will never do.

If you're not interested in shelling out the twenty bucks or so to have the original hem put back on, then the "cut and fray" is for you. Stand in front of the mirror, pick the length that's right for you, and throw a pin in for a marker. Take them off and mark a straight line with a ruler and a blue ballpoint pen a quarter-inch longer than your desired length. (Don't worry—the ink mark comes off in the wash.) Cut along the line, then fold the cut leg over, lining it up with the other leg, and repeat the cutting process. The fray comes into place only after washing and drying. There you are—the true definition of frugal, but with a terribly chic finish to boot.

Wear and Care

Most good-quality denim should shrink only in length, usually about a quarter of an inch. Eventually, many dryer loads later, they will shrink a bit in width, too. And you'll know if it's the dryer that's making them smaller or if it's just the result of that molten-chocolate cake you had with lunch. So be sure to consider the shrinkage factor when shopping.

real style secret

HOW TO KEEP DARK JEANS DARK

There's no getting around it. Over time, all things come to a fade. To keep your jeans darker longer, wash them less often. When you *do* launder them, follow these steps:

- Turn them inside out.
- Wash them in cold water with mild detergent and a quarter-cup of white vinegar.
- Air-dry them.

As an alternative measure, have them dry-cleaned. It will preserve the color longer than regular machine washing and drying will.

Have It Three Ways

The same pair of jeans can give you three completely different looks—daytime, office, and out on the town. All it takes is some creativity with accessories to get maximum flexibility out of one pair of jeans—amazing!

On casual days—when you're lunching with friends or hitting the mall or going to your kid's soccer game—team jeans with a T-shirt or tank, a zip hoody, and a pair of sneakers, sandals, or flip-flops. A belt is optional, especially if you have a good fit in the waist. In winter, add a cute fitted sweater and a pair of boots with a soft, unstructured shoulder bag to match.

To take your jeans to work, match them up with a tailored button-down shirt, a blazer, a belt, and a pair of leather loafers, flats, or pumps. Finish off the look with a scarf or piece of jewelry and a chic bucket bag.

To spruce them up for an evening out, wear them with your sexiest black top, a pair of gorgeous heels, and some killer earrings. Or pair them with a short, fitted, Chanel-type jacket, a lacy tank top, pearls, a clutch handbag, and stilettos. Accessorize them any way you would a pair of black dress pants—you'll love the look.

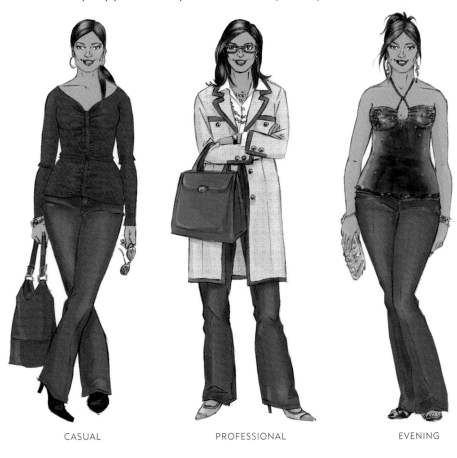

CASUAL   PROFESSIONAL   EVENING

CHAPTER 5

Detailing Your Style

ACCESSORIES

$\mathcal{S}$*ometimes, expressing your style* can be as easy as sporting a chic watch, carrying the right bag, or wearing a pair of shoes laced with attitude. You don't need to be a fashionista or spend a ton of money—you just need to know how to accessorize.

Clothing may make the man, but accessories definitely make the woman. I consider them to be the frosting on the cake of style, and they can speak volumes about your personality.

There should always be a balance between your wardrobe and your accessories. Otherwise, you run the risk of looking overstyled and exaggerated, or boring and forgettable. **This chapter will teach you the basics of accessorizing in a classic and beautiful way.** You'll learn what to invest in and how to maximize the potential of your best basics.

real style secret

THE SWITCH

If you regularly carry a shoulder bag, switch sides every so often to avoid throwing your shoulder line physically off balance. This is especially important for those of you who carry the equivalent of an anvil in your everyday purse. No amount of style is worth the discomfort of a sore neck and shoulder. You can take care of yourself *and* be stylish at the same time.

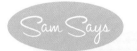

THE BAG OF THE MOMENT IS JUST THAT

Spending a lot of money on a hot, trendy bag? Be careful. Styles change faster than you can say "Louis Vuitton." You don't want to be caught dead toting last season's look when the magazines are gushing over something new. If you are willing to spend a fortune on a bag, make sure it's a classic that will look stylish for years to come.

Bags and Purses

The right bag can add a touch of sophistication to even the most casual outfit. Spending a bit more money on a few timeless bags is definitely the way to go. But if you don't have the dough, find a bag you love at a price that fits your budget.

Fashion did not create all bags equal. Your needs require different solutions, and the basics include bags for daytime and work.

Your daytime bags should be both casual and functional. Look for comfort and durability, and start your collection with neutral and versatile colors like black, camel, or brown.

Classic handbags come in many shapes and sizes. Which one is best suited to you hinges primarily on how you prefer to carry a bag and how much you need to put in it.

A clutch is streamlined and smart, and can go from day to night with ease. This is one of my favorites, because it is modern and classic at the same time. Styled like an envelope, a clutch is functional enough to hold all your basics. Just be sure you never overfill it, or you'll ruin its lines. Carry it in your hand, under your arm, or looped around your wrist if there's a strap attached.

A tote is casual and great for daytime. Available in many different sizes, it can hold a lot while giving you a sporty but feminine vibe. Ideally, a tote should be able to go from the hand to the shoulder with ease.

A shoulder bag is probably the easiest bag to carry, and it comes in a wide range of shapes. It is important to keep this bag in proportion to your body, because it rests close to it. Comfort is a consideration, too, so make sure the straps don't dig in and pinch. Your personal preferences will determine the length —ranging from just under the arm to low on the hip—but always remember to consider your height and choose wisely. A shorter woman can be dragged down by a long shoulder bag.

Backpacks can be found in a diversity of fabrics and sizes. This is not your kid's clunky school backpack, but, rather, a grown-up version that takes the weight of your bag off one side and completely frees up your hands and arms. The best backpacks are small and easy to access, so you don't have to undo a hundred pockets and toggles to get what you need. Choose feminine colors and sleek, refined styles that don't complicate your look.

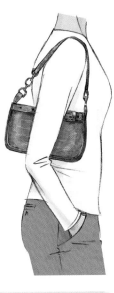

real style secret

THE POCHETTE—THE NEW "EVERYTHING BAG"

Pochette means "small pocket" in French, and that's exactly what this bag is. It has emerged as a sweeping trend that seems to be sticking around for a while, so it may behoove you to have one. This petite bag is normally less than twelve inches long, and typically has a zipper and a skinny strap. Use it for daytime when you're not going to carry a lot, and let it transition into a night out, tucked away under your shoulder. You'll love how easy it is to carry. Almost every designer is making one, so check out a pochette the next time you're at the mall and feel like practicing your French.

The handbag is meant to be carried, as the name implies, in your hand. This bag is ladylike and sophisticated even in its most casual incarnations. I also find it very chic when carried in the bend of your arm, showcased like a work of art.

Bucket bags usually have a rounded bottom, and are the novelty version of a tote bag. They can be a bit dressier than a basic tote, and actually do resemble a bucket in a way. Just don't go overboard and fill yours up like one.

The fabric of your handbag is just as important as the style. The choice you make will dictate when and how you can carry each bag, so keep these common fabrics in mind when shopping.

Leather is the consummate fabric for a bag, getting better with age and capable of enduring just about anything.

Patent leather is leather's naughty sibling. Shiny and strong, it's an attention-getter that works well for a hot night out, or during the day in a brighter, more casual color. It's best to add patent leather to your collection only when all the basics are in place.

Canvas is the way to go when you want a sturdy, casual bag. Because it can take the weight, it serves well as a bookbag, tote, or messenger bag. It's perfect for the beach, and—best of all—it's washable.

Even the most exclusive bag designers in the world offer versions made of nylon or some form of microfiber. If you are prone to spilling your espresso or if you live in a rainy climate, you can't go wrong with a lightweight and strong nylon bag.

A satin bag is sleek and dressy, and can be carried in the daytime if it's mixed with other fabrics. The soft sheen beautifully complements any fabric you're wearing.

Suede, reserved exclusively for fall and winter, lets you change with the seasons. It offers a textured sophistication while maintaining the solid sturdiness you find in its sister fabric, grain leather.

Specialty skins—such as crocodile, alligator, lizard, python, and pony hair—reek of status and wealth, and can add a luxurious statement to your handbag collection.

Jewelry

Jewelry is like a rite of passage for a girl. There is something magical and almost ritualistic about a female adorning herself with precious metals and gems to look and feel beautiful. You should wear jewelry not only for others but for yourself. It makes you feel special, and it becomes a part of you.

A piece of jewelry can do all the talking for both you and what you're wearing. You don't need much to be stylish—just a few strategically placed baubles. If you can afford the real deal—terrific. If not, there's nothing wrong with buying well-made copies of the good stuff. Nobody needs to know but you, your best friend, and . . . okay . . . me.

Though gorgeous jewelry trends will come and go, there are a few classic pieces that remain timeless in their beauty. Following are a few essentials that should be in the top drawer of your jewelry box.

Diamond stud earrings are a classic that can complete your look no matter how you're dressed or where you are. Whether you are working out at the gym or shmoozing at an elegant cocktail party, diamond studs always look beautiful. They are simple and feminine, and they will never do you wrong.

A few pairs of simple hoop earrings can keep you fashionable in almost any situation. They're fine for both day and night, and the size will determine the look you get. They can be conservative little hoops that hug the earlobe, or larger ones that give you an urban-sexy look. Try a medium one for everyday, and add drama with a sparkling one for evening.

A strand or two of pearls and a pair of pearl earrings are ladylike and classy. They are definitely thought of as more conservative, and though your favorite magazines will make them a trend from time to time, no one will ever argue with their feminine beauty and essential place in fashion history.

Nothing beats a diamond tennis bracelet as arm candy. It's understated yet elegant, and as far as I'm concerned, you could put one on and never take it off. It's clearly the solution for any event, and it layers beautifully with other jewelry.

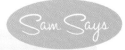
Sam Says

JEWELRY IS A SENTIMENTAL JOURNEY

When a piece of jewelry is worn for a long time, it can absorb some of your energy and history, becoming a very powerful component of your style. In this way, jewelry has extraordinary sentimental value when passed down from one person to another.

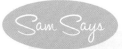

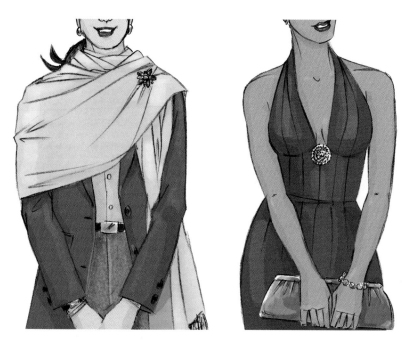

GET ODD WITH BROOCHES

Brooches should always be worn in odd numbers: a single pin or a group of three. (Five is pushing it just a bit.) Two pins together can look too balanced and contrived, so the asymmetry of three smaller brooches is much more appealing.

A jeweled brooch is a basic that adds a bit of dazzle to everything. Pin one on a T-shirt or a tank top, a dress or a denim jacket. In fact, I challenge you to find a place where it doesn't look good. It can be sexy when pinned to the center of a strapless dress and looks cool on the waistband of your jeans or clipped in your hair when you're wearing it up. And it's elegant when used to fasten a scarf into place or to join a few strands of pearls. Whether you want to make a subtle statement or catch someone's eye in a major way, you can always rely on the brooch.

An everyday watch is a staple that serves dual purposes—fashion and function. A beautiful watch can be all the jewelry you need on any given day. Decide on the strap according to your personality. If you are more casual, leather or some kind of variation is for you. If you tend to wear more jewelry on a regular basis, then a bracelet band in gold or silver will be a better choice. Select it based on the color of the jewelry you wear most often.

You don't have to be married to have diamond or cubic zirconia (CZ) eternity bands on your finger. They are wonderful when stacked in multiples or layered with other rings, providing a striking frame or backdrop for almost any style.

Cocktail rings are a bit more dramatic, with a flourish that makes them special. Go for a look that's interesting and fun without being too garish or gaudy. Most over-the-top rings will end up looking fake—even if they're not. Have fun playing with different-colored stones and mixing things up a bit. True to their name, cocktail rings are shown off beautifully when you're holding a drink, and they add some pizzazz and sparkle to your favorite evening looks. So keep them there, in the evening, where they belong.

A thin gold or silver chain is wonderful in its simplicity, and can be worn against skin or fabric. It can bring a slight bit of detail and attention to the neckline, and can be worn by women of any age. A charm necklace adds a little more interest. Keep the size of the charm in proportion to your shoulders and neckline—not too big, not too small. You don't want it to look like it's a speck floating in the ocean or a boulder competing with your face.

The length of the chain is also important. Use the charm as your guide, and keep it centered between the bottom of your neck and the top of your bustline. Or let it fall into the hollow at the base of your neck. Whatever you do, don't wear it so long that it plunges—perhaps never to be seen again—into your cleavage.

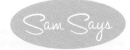

Sam Says

GO BEYOND THE BASICS

Jewelry can be playful and fun, so throw on some of these nonessentials when you want to bump things up a bit. An oversized bangle on the wrist provides a great individual focal point, as does an exaggerated earring that brings the focus to your face. Layering necklaces—a charm with a choker, or a few chains in varying lengths and thicknesses—can fill out your neckline and give you a bohemian-chic vibe.

Your local thrift store is one of the best places to find interesting, one-of-a-kind jewelry. Delve into the styles of the past, and mix and match your vintage finds with your best pieces. Originality is key in choosing your accessories, and will set your sense of style apart from everyone else's.

Not Your Everyday Shoes

There's an old saying: "People always look at your shoes." What better reason to learn how to wear them well?

You can brighten the most ordinary outfit in the world when you put some effort into the shoes you wear. Remember—though fabulous shoes can add flash to the most inexpensive dress, cheap shoes can tear down even a costly designer ensemble.

We have already covered shoe basics in Chapter 3, and now it's time for some fun. Shoes are the one accessory almost every body type can enjoy with little or no effort. Once you understand the variations of color, pattern, texture, fabric, and print, you can start to filter in some specialty shoes that will take your feet out of the box. Here are a few styles that can add some punch and distinction.

THE SPECIALTY SHOE	THE WHAT	THE HOW
Stilettos	A skinny higher heel, two and a half inches and up, with a pointy toe. They make the pump look tame by comparison. The more colorful and outrageous, the better.	Wear them to spice up an all-black ensemble, so your sexy stilettos become the focal point. Excellent with dark denim, a cropped evening gaucho pant, or a shorter skirt. A must with a sleek clutch.
Primary-colored pumps	A rounded toe or a soft point, with a heel up to three inches. Your color choice makes it special. Red, pink, green, or turquoise—be creative.	Great for day or night when you want to make a splash. Choose color tones by the seasons. Sweet with a denim mini or a daytime dress topped off with a jean jacket.
Animal prints (real or faux)	Mock-crocodile, lizard, python, leopard, or zebra. Looks great in a pump, stiletto, boot, or sandal.	Contrasts dressy with casual when worn with jeans. Exclusive and confident with a suit. Textural and dramatic with your evening looks.

THE SPECIALTY SHOE	THE WHAT	THE HOW
Metallic leather	Darker tones of gold, silver, pewter, bronze, or copper work best in the fall. Lighter metallics smolder in the summer sun. Best in a strappy heel or sandal.	A great alternative to black, nude, or brown when dressing up your dresses. Flashy but sophisticated. Excellent for hard-to-match dress colors like navy, green, purple, and fuchsia.
Suede	The reverse side of leather that is buffed velvety smooth. Rich and elegant, but for the fall and winter only. Choose tones like burgundy, hunter, chocolate, camel, pumpkin, and fuchsia.	Beautiful with office separates like a tweed pant and cashmere knit. Excellent in a boot when paired with tights and a mini. Rugged and sexy when worn with jeans and a cable-knit sweater.
Patent leather	Shiny and vampy, with a hard, glossy surface. Best in pumps, strappy high heels, stilettos, sandals, and flats.	A strong statement with a suit or an evening tuxedo. Chic and relaxed in a pointy flat. Dresses up a sundress as a shiny sandal in a bright color.
Strappy sandals	With slender heels at least two inches high, and thin, intersecting straps of leather. Perfect for summer days and nights.	Wear them with jeans rolled up with a double-wide cuff to the length of capris, and with every style of summer dress. Just don't ever wear them with hosiery.
Wedges	With a four-inch heel, usually made of cork, and a graduated wedge to the toe for extra balance, this is everyone's leg-lengthening staple in summer.	Wedges make the half-pint a whole pint. A moderate wedge will give you a leggy look when your pants cover them up a bit, and when you wear them with capris, a mini, or a low-slung skirt.
Espadrilles	Usually fashioned in canvas, with a flat or wedged heel and the sides of the sole wrapped in jute rope. Sometimes secured with an ankle strap for support.	Summery and sweet. Pair them with a flowing A-line skirt, shorts, a sundress, or an old pair of jeans.
Cowboy boots	Though they tend to come and go as a fashion trend, cowboy boots are always in style. Keep a special pair tucked away in your closet.	Buy them in a wild fun color or skin, or play it safe and stick with a neutral. Wear them with vintage denim and a corduroy blazer, or with a jean skirt and tank top. Don't forget the belt and a cool buckle.

When I was young, my mom always bought shoes to match her bag. She had a closet stacked with extraordinary purses and the shoes to accompany them. I was fascinated by this notion, and just assumed it was what every woman did.

These days, you don't have to be so rigidly matched. I still love the idea, because, when it comes to fashion and style, I'm a bit of a purist. But for the modern woman, it's okay to loosen things up. I encourage you to be creative and have some fun here. Pair a dressy shoe with a casual bag, and vice versa. As long as the theme between the shoe and bag is in line—such as color, pattern, or texture—you're fine. You'll have two accessories that complement each other but can still stand on their own.

REFINING YOUR FOOTWEAR

Are you one of those girls who has spent obscene amounts of money acquiring all the right shoes? Your closet is a shrine, housing the crème de la crème of footwear. Your dilemma? A few of your favorites have been worn to death and are in dire need of some freshening up—a shoe lift, if you will. Where to turn, what to do?

THE BEST TIME TO SHOE-SHOP

Did you know that there is a right and a wrong time of day to go shopping for shoes? Throughout the day, your feet naturally swell and grow a bit in size, sometimes expanding a full size by the end of the day. So the best time to shop for shoes is midday, when you're somewhere in the middle of the swelling cycle. However, if you are buying an evening shoe that you know you'll wear only at night, it is best to shop later in the day. This way, you are almost guaranteed a comfortable fit, and you won't have to kick off your shoes under the dinner table because of the swelling and pain.

Check out your local cobbler. You'd be amazed at the tricks that can be performed on footwear you're ready to give up on. So, before you throw away a pair of good shoes that seem to be on their last leg, see your shoe guy for a quick fix. From reviving to reinventing, he is the tailor for your footwear.

If your shoes are scuffed, if the leather is faded, if that creamy satin heel has turned to a dirty beige, you can refresh them by getting them redyed. Your shoe professional can bring most leather, suede, and fabric back to life. You can even change the color after you've gotten your fill of the original one. Just remember,

real style secret

DANCE RUBBER

All of Hollywood's stylists and celebrities rely on dance rubber. It's a thin piece of rubber that is textured to prevent slipping. It is glued to the bottom of a shoe with heavy-duty rubber cement. The dance rubber gives you a strong grip that can boost your confidence when you're sporting even the highest pair of heels.

You can buy an inexpensive peel-and-stick version at the drugstore and apply it on your own. It usually comes in black or gray, so don't worry about trying to match it to the sole of your shoe. After all, this trick is more about practicality than style. If you prefer, you can have a cobbler apply a higher-quality version, in which case the color can usually be matched perfectly.

under most circumstances, you can go only from lighter to darker tones when making such a change.

If you're like me and you wear your shoes very hard, don't stress. They can be resoled in a snap—inside and out—by your cobbler.

Need a little extra something in your shoes for comfort? You can opt to buy inexpensive padding at your local drugstore, which is fine and dandy. Or you can have your cobbler insert some under the inside leather sole of your shoe for a more subtle approach. Most people joke about lifts, but for the half-pint, this is serious business. You have two options here: You can stack up the height by adding layers of leather to the heel and sole of the shoe, or you can have a lift put into the shoe. Lifts can add a couple of inches—just be sure you're comfortable in them and they don't make your back hurt. If you have second thoughts down the road, most lifts can be removed.

Scarves

A lovely, flowing scarf will always be a symbol of femininity—sometimes even of status—and will add depth and dimension to any outfit. These days, scarves come in a variety of sizes and fabrics—from sporty cottons to elegant silks, from practical polyester to indulgent cashmere—so they can be worn every day of the year. There's no limit to their versatility, as they can be used for anything from a head wrap to a hip wrap—and a whole lot in between.

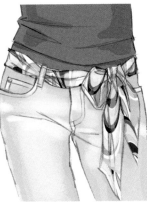

Anyone can wear a scarf as an accessory—as long as you consider your neckline. If you run a little short in the neck, or if your neck is lean, narrower scarves are for you. If you have a fuller neck, a scarf that is wide—yet thin and lightweight—will balance you out. Avoid wrapping it around your neck, which will add extra bulk. Instead, drape it around your neck to add levels to your outfit and hide a fuller bust in the process. If your neck is long and swanlike, wrap the scarf around a couple of times for coverage and added fullness.

real style **secret**

SCARVES UNLIMITED

The only limit to the ways in which you can wear a scarf is your imagination. Just take a look at all your options:

- Tie a colorful printed scarf to the strap of a handbag.
- Wear an oversized one as an evening wrap.
- Use a scarf as a belt by weaving a narrow one through the loops of your favorite pants or jeans. You can let the ends hang free, tie them in a knot or bow, or tuck them under for a more finished look.
- Wear one in your hair as a head wrap or to finish a ponytail.
- Tuck a small one in a lapel pocket.
- Fold a large, square scarf on an angle and tie it around your hips to camouflage broadness. This trick also works if you have no hips, because it will create visual interest. Hip hips—hooray!

Belts

The waistline is one of the hottest places to express your individuality with an interesting detail. Look for belts with embellishments—such as studs, grommets, and other metallic treatments—and weathered, vintage styles that are textured or embossed. They add a unique touch and tie an outfit together, and—yes—some women even use them to hold up their pants. Belts can give you a waistline where you have none, and can finish the look of a skirt, dress, pants, or jeans as a great accessory should.

A thick belt draws attention to your waistline, so it has the ability to minimize fuller hips. A skinny one suits short-waisted women, because it defines the waist without overwhelming it. It also says subtle and conservative, making it smart for the corporate environment.

A belt with a detailed or oversized buckle is sexy, rugged, and boyish, and it's hot with denim. A chain belt is very feminine and looks terrific with skirts. Think jewelry for your waist. A sash is cute with dresses, and can be worn in either a matching or contrasting color.

real style secret

INSTANT BELTS FOR SMALL BUCKS

Build your own belt with a buckle, some fabric, and your imagination. Find a buckle you like at a notions store—a metal or plastic one that fastens without the need for holes. Just weave a scarf, piece of fabric, or length of ribbon through the buckle, and you have a belt that can be customized for any outfit.

Thread some two-inch ribbon—sleek satin or textured grosgrain—through your belt loops and tie it in a bow on your side for a fun, flirty look.

Eyeglasses and Sunglasses

Knowing what eyewear is right for you starts with knowing the shape of your face. Just like you identified your body type in Chapter 1, it's time to face your face. To determine its shape, grab an eyeliner pencil or a tube of lipstick and hit the bathroom mirror. You'll have to get close up and shut one eye. Trace an outline of your face directly onto the mirror. Step back and check it out: your face shape, plain as day. (Sorry about having to get the makeup off your mirror—I never claimed to be an expert in cleanup.)

Generally, we all fall into one of five categories: oblong, oval, round, heart-shaped, and square. Your face shape tells you which glasses are best for you, as outlined in the chart on page 110.

While sunglasses protect your eyes, they are as much a part of your wardrobe as any accessory. Some women even collect the perfect sunglasses the same way they stock up on fine jewelry—and some eyewear can cost just as much.

Experiment with frame colors like dark navy, hunter green, and rich purple. Try textures like tortoise, brushed metallics, and mother-of-pearl. Or play it safe with plain old black. Lens colors should be selected based on your skin tone and hair color.

Your sunglasses say as much about your personality as your favorite shoes or best pair of jeans, and are a major component of style. You can wear them on your head like a stylish headband, hide behind them when you feel like avoiding the world, or just wear 'em when you need 'em to avoid the squint factor. Whatever the case, have fun with your glasses—these year-round accessories aren't just for the sun anymore. In fact, they're fabulous in the winter with a scarf and a chic piece of outerwear.

You'll find that buying glasses or sunglasses is much like choosing your clothing. You need to keep things in proportion, flatter your face shape with styles that can play visual tricks, and select what looks and feels best for you.

FACE SHAPE	FACIAL CHARACTERISTICS	BEST GLASSES
Oblong	Longer than it is wide, and narrow from the top of the forehead to the chin—like a rectangle with rounded edges	Try frames that have a top-to-bottom depth. Decorative or contrasting temples ("arms" on the sides of glasses) will add width to the face.
Oval	Considered to be the most desirable and proportionate face shape, with a narrower chin and higher cheekbones	Wear frames that are as wide as, or wider than, the broadest part of your face. Keep their overall size in balance with the size of your face, and almost any frame will work.
Round	A fuller face, with no angles	Choose rectangles and squares to provide contrast, or cat-eye frames that add visual lift. A wider frame is always a plus, and can make your chin appear more defined. Look for temples ("arms" on the side of glasses) that attach a bit higher up on the frame for extra definition. Avoid round frames.
Heart	A wider forehead, high cheekbones, and a narrow, pointy chin	Opt for rimless frames or those in a lighter tone. Frames that are fuller at the bottom, such as aviators, will fill out your face, as will butterfly styles. You also have the face shape to carry an oversized frame. Do I see Jackie O sunglasses in your future?
Square	A broad forehead, a wider jaw and chin, with cheekbones to match	Narrow, oval frames with temples ("arms" on the side of glasses) that attach at the middle of the lens and those that sit higher on your face are best to offset your jawline. Round frames and those with some curve work well to provide contrast.

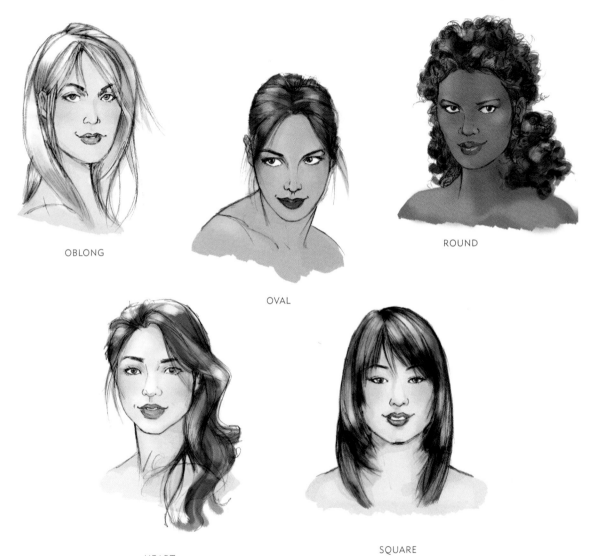

OBLONG

OVAL

ROUND

HEART

SQUARE

CHAPTER 6

The Corporate Runway

DRESSING FOR
THE *NEW* WORKPLACE

Do you sometimes show up at work feeling as if **everyone in the office received a memo on how to dress the part but you?** Do you gaze around and wonder why your co-workers seem to look and feel so comfortable, even fashionable, yet you look like you're about to audition for the part of the corporate female in an eighties movie?

The new workplace has broken a lot of the old rules, and keeping pace with the new ones can present a real challenge. The stiff, professional look that prevailed for so long is beginning to soften, and though "professional" is still the order of the day, "stiff" is no longer on the agenda. Today's office environment allows you to be corporate, casual, and comfortable—all at the same time. **It's called dressing for success in the *new* workplace, and it's not as hard as you may think.**

A woman's femininity is one of her strongest assets in the workplace. So I say use it, and use it well. A woman who has confidence and expresses it through her sense of style is a force to be reckoned with. You

When shopping for a
suit pant, stay away
from cuffed pants
unless you have legs
for days. Uncuffed
pants add length to
your legs; cuffs cut
them off. The
horizontal line of the
cuff stops the eye and
makes legs appear
shorter. If you are a
willow or a taller
diamond, cuffs are
okay and a matter of
preference.

know exactly who she is when she walks into a room, and her look commands
enough attention for three men. This is real power dressing, and it can be extraor-
dinarily effective.

It is true that most work clothing for women is inspired by menswear. This is the
source of dressing for success for the professional female, and it was a major trend
in the eighties. The yuppie woman felt she needed to dress in a more masculine way
to be competitive in the corporate arena, and back then, she was probably right.

Though donning a suit every day is still de rigueur for some women, there is
no denying the fact that looks and styles have changed. Today, the important
things are the elements that *separate* the women from the good ol' boys, and
that's what this chapter is all about—being a woman at work, not a woman in
men's clothing. If your professional environment demands that you go corporate
all the way, every day, it's easy to comply without becoming the victim of a hos-
tile takeover of your sense of style.

How to Buy the Right Suit

If you have a designer brand that you've come to rely on for fit and style in your
casual clothing, find out if the company makes suits, too. If so, that's the first
place to start. If not, consider your budget and do some research. You can spend
a fortune on one exceptional suit that you'll wear every so often, or you can buy
a few less expensive ones that you'll wear more regularly. Your professional needs
will dictate which path to follow.

Know what you are shopping for before you leave the house. Is this suit purchase an update of your old standby that's on its last leg? Is it an upgrade to
something better and more special because now you have a clearer understanding of what looks good on you? Is it an addition to your basic suits, a novelty version to break up the norm? Or are you a suit virgin? Whatever the case, have a
specific idea in mind so you can tailor this shopping trip to your particular needs
and avoid getting sidetracked.

The most critical component of a suit is the cut. Look for feminine lines that will set your suit apart from your man's. Because suits are generally thought of as menswear, make sure to counter that idea as often as possible when you shop for one.

Select jackets whose shapes are defined with darts and tapers. Seek out feminine lines such as narrower arms, slightly padded shoulders, tapered waists, and a plunging gorge, which is the V on the jacket that is surrounded by the lapel. A deeper gorge affords a more feminine look.

Choose a lapelled jacket that flatters your shoulder line. If you have weak shoulders, a peaked lapel, which has a pronounced upward point, brings attention where you need it. A notched lapel has a downward point and a small triangular cutout. It's best for broad shoulders, because it draws the eye away from the shoulder line. A shawl collar is rounded and soft with no hard lines at all, and is a flattering way to diminish a strong shoulder line.

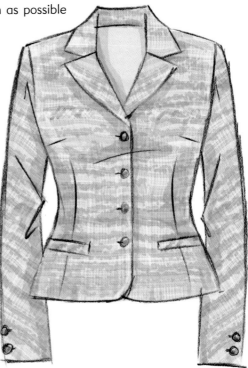

real style secret

BUTTONING UP

When you find a suit jacket or blazer that seems to be just right, do one last thing before buying it—take the button/zipper test. If for any reason you can't button or zip the jacket fully—or if it's too tight when you do—you must seriously reconsider making the purchase. Even if you have no intention of ever doing it up, the time will inevitably come when you'll try. Then you'll hear my voice in the back of your mind chanting, "I told you so."

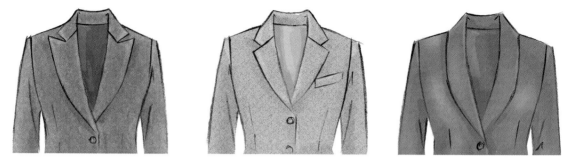

PEAKED   NOTCHED   SHAWL

Your suit jacket can also be boxy, with no lapel or collar, buttoning up to the neck with a clean, scooped neckline. Or it can be tapered, with a small lapel just around the collar. Both of these options are very feminine.

You'll have to decide whether you prefer a one-, two-, or three-button jacket or a double-breasted one. Single-button is the most classic and common style for women. It works beautifully in a longer length, which can help to minimize hips. The V of a one-button jacket also minimizes a fuller bust.

Two- or three-button jackets give you coverage when you want to appear more conservative. Two buttons work well in any length, and three buttons are best in fitted, shorter styles that stop at the waist. However, if you're looking to minimize your hips, a longer three-button jacket that skims over them is fine.

In my opinion, double-breasted suit jackets work well only as a lady's tuxedo. They are a bit dated for the workplace, so try to avoid them except for dressy work events or as evening wear.

Suit pants will often be sold separately, and may be available in different styles to fit different body types. You may also be able to find a pantsuit with a skirt as an option, in which case you should buy both. Sometimes you can even buy a three-piece set, which includes the jacket, skirt, and pants. Lucky, lucky, lucky.

Your pant style will be either flat-front or pleated, and a flat front is always more sleek looking. Choose low- or high-waisted styles, depending on your body type. Choose between a straight and a flared leg. The flared bottom is a wonderful contrast to the masculine styling of a suit jacket, so give it a try. If your body type says otherwise, a straight leg works just as well. You can even try a fuller, palazzo style.

The right skirt can enhance the look of your suit. Knee-length is the best option, and pencil is the best style. The high-waisted version, a throwback to the forties, gives you a fashionable and professional look and is best with a top tucked in. The low-waisted skirt is easy and basic.

Whichever option you prefer, the skirt should fall clean and straight, with a back or side zipper for a smoother fit. The idea here is always to look for a way to dress more femininely at work. A skirt with a slit, a fluted bottom, or a kick pleat will do the job nicely.

Next, think about color. A suit is best in a basic color—black, brown, navy, khaki, or gray—that will go with almost anything. If this is your first suit, buy it in black to be both versatile and safe. If this is a novelty addition, a nonneutral color is okay—as long as you don't get trapped by it. For example, a bold color like red can be too strong, and way too memorable. Instead, choose a more subtle shade like blush, which is somewhere between a beige and a pink, or khaki green. These colors are easy to work with, and are fun, feminine, and office-appropriate.

The fabric you select is important, so you should look for one that is comfortable and breathable. Most suiting is made from fine wool, or a blend of wool and other fabrics, such as viscose, which is a type of rayon. Wool is my number-one recommendation, since its durability will outperform most other fabrics in the workplace, and its many variations—including tropical-weight wool—make it a good all-season choice. A sturdy cotton twill is a nice alternative, especially in the warmest months or climates. Linen is also a good option when the temperature rises—if you can handle the wrinkle factor. (And let's face it, ladies, linen is going to wrinkle even if you never sit down and even if you keep your breathing to a minimum. It's the nature of the beast, so accept it or leave it on the rack.)

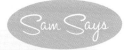

Avoid 100-percent polyester whenever possible. Even though it's easy to care for and rarely wrinkles, there are downsides to wearing an unnatural fabric. For example, if you happen to stand in the sun, it will glow with an unworldly shine and make you feel as if you're in a sweatbox. A poly blend is acceptable, but should not be your first choice.

The texture of the fabric can distinguish a suit to make it more interesting. Herringbone has a V-pattern woven through it in long vertical lines, which are alternately reversed to create a pattern. It is conservative, proper, and extremely suitworthy.

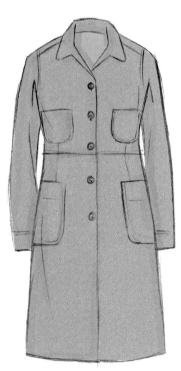
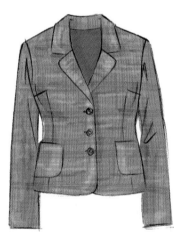
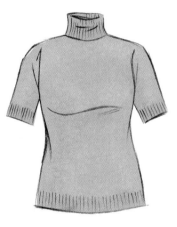

MIX-AND-MATCH SEPARATES

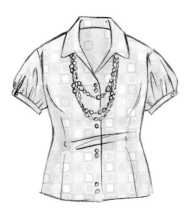
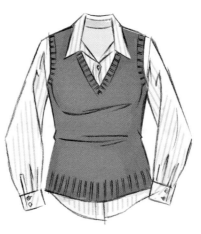
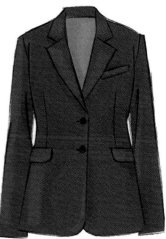
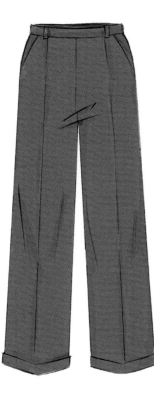
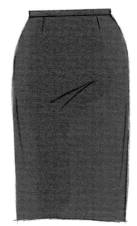
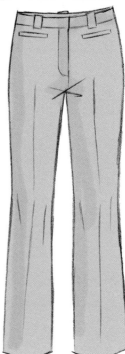

Q I always hear about gabardine in reference to suits. Is it some sort of fabric?

A Gabardine is not a fabric at all, but, rather, a type of weave. It is very sturdy, with a distinctive diagonal rib, and can be cotton, synthetic, or wool. Wool gabardine is beautiful and wears exceptionally well, hence its popularity. But gabardine in any fabric is equally appealing and rich looking.

A houndstooth weave has a pattern that forms a four-pointed star, and is often found in black and white. It is fine for a suit when the pattern is scaled down, but larger patterns are better worn one piece at a time, and paired with a solid color to break things up.

Tweed is my favorite of the textured fabrics, because it is so classy and sophisticated. Coco Chanel made the woman's tweed suit fashionable decades ago, and it is still a staple of the stylish businesswoman. Tweed has several shades of colored wool running through the fabric, giving it a characteristic flecked appearance. It is nubby and dense, and comes in a variety of weights. Tweed is a standout in the fall, so save it for September and beyond.

Next, consider the three Ps: pinstripes, plaids, and prints. These patterns can go to the office with you, as long as they have a feminine touch. The pinstripes, for example, can be pink on black instead of the classic white. The plaid can be a bit bolder than a typical menswear plaid, with some pretty colors—such as soft purples and greens—running through it. And prints—well, you're not likely to see a man in a printed suit unless you're watching old Elton John videos, so these are all girl, all the way. In most cases, the print is woven right into the fabric, and is tone-on-tone in color. Look for subtle prints here that whisper rather than shout.

Q I just landed an interview for my dream job, and I have been out of the office environment for a while. What can I wear that will look professional?

A Dressing for a job interview has changed a bit, but the rules remain the same. Keep it simple and professional, and retain a bit of personal style to set you apart from the competition. It is always better to be a bit overdressed rather than underdressed. It shows that you take the meeting and the job seriously. Wear a suit, or opt for a blazer with pants or a skirt. Team your outfit with high heels, which will correct slouching posture and give the impression of confidence and power.

Personalize your look with some simple jewelry and accessories. A pin on your lapel, a beautiful scarf, or some pretty earrings work fine. Perfume can be distracting—and even offensive to some—so I advise you to save it for date night.

The idea behind a job interview is to be yourself—and that includes your choice in clothing. If the outfit is stiff and tedious, that's how you'll come across. So think things through carefully, and you'll land the job with grace and style.

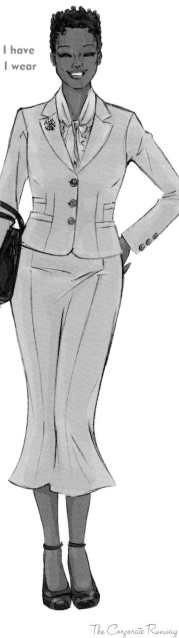

Accessorizing Your Suit

Now that you have some idea of how to shop for a suit, let's see how changing your accessories can give you a multitude of different looks from one simple foundation.

Like a man's suit, a woman's suit is a blank canvas. Whereas men have only shirts and ties to add personality and color, women have tops, accessories, and shoes to work with. So who do you think is going to win the race to the top of the corporate fashion ladder in the style department? Exactly!

Different tops will change the look of your suit, so always have at least three or four for every suit you own. Button-downs, camisoles, tanks, dressy Ts, and knits will all work beautifully to vary a classic suit.

If you're a true fan of the white shirt, bump it up the fashion ladder by playing with collars. Larger collars open up and frame your face, especially when pulled out and worn over the lapel of your jacket. Smaller collars are sweeter and more feminine, neatly tucked away under the lapel. A higher-necked collar is conservative, and a banded collar—such as a mandarin—provides a casual, airy look. You should never again think of a white shirt as plain. The options are truly endless, especially for the workplace.

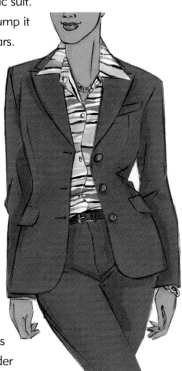

Instead of always taking the safe route with a basic white shirt or top, try one in a bright, rich color that will spice things up. Color has energy and can speak volumes about who you are. A jewel-toned shirt under a neutral-colored suit adds a dramatic focal point. A shirt in a muted tone provides a wash of color for interest, without being too bold and imposing. You get the idea.

When you're ready to break away from the predictable, add pattern and personality to your suit with a printed top. Bold stripes, swirls of color, and strong patterns will take your look from conservative to creative in a flash.

To soften a suit's masculine lines, team it with a sleek satin camisole that features a lacy décolletage, or a silk blouse open to your cleavage. Try a fitted tank with some piping, a blousy tube top, or a sexy knit that shows your curves. All will do the trick nicely.

Scarves, like a knockout tie on a man, can add real personality to a suit. Try a small, patterned one spilling out of your breast pocket, or tuck a large, printed one under your lapel. Wear a short scarf instead of a necklace, or tie a long one around the waist of a pencil skirt. Wrap an oversized wool or cashmere scarf around your shoulders instead of a coat, and fasten it with a pin.

Shoes are always terrific attention-getters, and few things are more beautiful than a woman in a suit accented with a heel. Pair a creamy suit with a brightly colored pointy heel for a bit of dazzle. Try a straitlaced gray suit with a pink pump to make you both soft and serious at the same time. Knock 'em dead with alligator or mock-crocodile stilettos teamed with textured tights and a sophisticated tweed number.

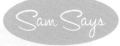

Sam Says

ADD SOME POP WITH A PATTERN

A beautiful pant or skirt and a simple blouse paired with a three-quarter-length printed jacket will make you the envy of your floor. Talk about first impressions! Wear the jacket as a coat, and let it do all the talking for you at the beginning and the end of the workday. Color, geometrics, and—wow!—they all combine to turn a few heads.

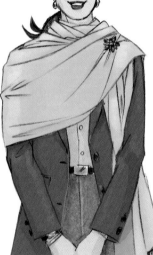

Are you still wondering what to do with all that jewelry you've been collecting over the years? Well, you have five days a week and a plain suit to work with.

In the office, the basics will always score some points. In the *new* workplace, they'd better be touchdowns. A suit can handle a stronger piece of jewelry, but the key to jewelry in the office is to keep it conservative. Though the pieces can be bold, they must also be clean and uncomplicated.

Think primary jewel tones to add a punch of color. A stone without too many flashy facets works best. I love a cabochon ring or pin for the office. These gems are polished, smooth, and rounded with no facets at all, which makes them subtler.

Pearls, of course, are a must. Classic off-white ones are fine, but try some colors like champagne, pale pink, gray, and brown. A white shirt open at the neck with a strand of pearls is rich and commanding.

Try a pin on your lapel to draw attention to an otherwise plain suit. Layer a few thin bracelets in gold, silver, or semiprecious stones on your wrist to keep things stylish. When your jacket comes off at lunch, you'll be serving fashion in a beautiful way. Finally, a classic watch with a bracelet or leather band is the quintessential work accessory, and is worth the investment. Choose one that is professional yet graceful and feminine. It will speak volumes about your style, and may be the only accessory your wrist will need.

real style secret

THE PANTYHOSE ALTERNATIVE

If you hate to wear pantyhose but need to have a refined look with a skirt or dress in the office, tanned legs can replace nude hose beautifully. The world of self-tanners evolves a notch every day. From self-tanning lotions and tinted moisturizers to spray-on tans and aerosol tans in a can, there's an option for everyone. Always exfoliate first for the best results.

Q I work in an office, and I have to haul a lot of files back and forth every day. Is there a bag I can carry that will hold it all, but still look tidy and professional?

A Practical and stylish really can go hand in hand. Your workbag should be as fabulous as your best handbag, and also be large enough to hold your purse and your papers. Think lightweight, comfortable, and accommodating, with an air of corporate respectability. You don't want to tote a huge bag that looks as if you just packed for a day at the beach with kids. I recommend two bags for use in the business arena: the messenger bag and the portfolio.

The messenger bag features a large flap and an adjustable shoulder strap. It is most commonly found in canvas, nylon, and microfiber. Stick to a dark neutral color, such as black, gray, navy, or brown.

The portfolio is the woman's version of the classic briefcase. It is usually fashioned out of soft, supple leather, with clean, elegant lines that are as feminine as you are.

For the label conscious, there are workbags styled by top-name designers, and this is where you can spend some hard-earned cash. Not only do you get your money's worth by carrying it five days a week, but you also let others know that you value your work enough to dress it for success.

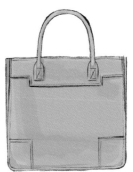

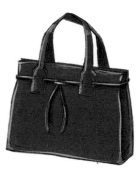

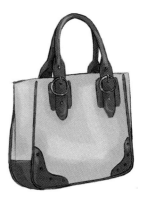

WORKBAGS

After all I've said about suits, I want you to be aware that it's not necessary to wear one every day. Even in the power-dressed corporate arena, you can break out of the mold and take advantage of the many skirt and dress options.

The power of a suit is diluted when you wear one day in and day out. So feel free to mix things up a little, experimenting with separates and injecting some real style into your everyday looks. And save the suit for when you have a major client meeting or presentation and want to present yourself as a don't-mess-with-me authority figure.

Q **I'm not a "suit" person. What else can I wear to the office that's dressy and professional?**

A A beautiful tailored dress will work nicely for the office, especially if it's paired with an elegant high-heeled pump or boot. Confine it to a conservative color or muted pattern, and add interest with a scarf or jewelry.

Skirt-and-blouse and pant-and-blouse combinations also have enormous potential and flexibility. Whether you buy separates or simply play with pieces of your favorite suits, you can get endless looks by mixing and matching.

Casual Fridays

The popular office trend of casual Fridays is spilling into Mondays through Thursdays, too, as many companies ease up on their definition of proper business attire. This is your opportunity to step out of the cubicle and bring some of your individuality to work with you.

Khaki pants or khaki skirts are ideal choices for an office that has relaxed the dress code. They've emerged as a workplace favorite because they blend a casual look with a professional one. As comfortable as a pair of jeans but dressier —no wonder khakis are a staple in most uniforms around the country.

Pair your khaki pants or skirt with an easy top, like a knit, a long-sleeved T, or a crisp button-down shirt. Since khakis are plain, your choice in tops shouldn't be. Have some fun here, experimenting with a printed top, a T-shirt and a fitted jacket, or a cute knit vest and button-down shirt.

A simple skirt, top, and novelty shoe, when done right, can be very professional yet still fall within the casual realm. Wear a pencil skirt with a button-down shirt tucked in, then step into a special shoe for flair.

When you want to take more of a risk—like wearing jeans to work—make sure they are darker denim so they'll resemble a dress pant. You should always be respectful of your work environment, especially if you have a high-level job. In some office environments, jeans are simply not appropriate, so make sure you have the blessing of the human-resources department before showing up in them.

Every day, your office provides the opportunity for you to make a statement with your sense of style. The choices are endless, and they can all fit in with what your employer deems to be appropriate professional attire. Don't be afraid to take a few risks and experiment with your work wardrobe. Then take your own stroll down the corporate runway.

FOLLOW THE LEADERS

An effective way to judge what is acceptable to wear to work on a casual Friday is to look to your superiors. They set the tone in the workplace, including dressing and style. If they are dressed up and professional even when allowed to take a more casual approach, chances are they want you to follow suit. If they hold out all week, then happily show up in their favorite jeans and loafers every Friday, odds are you can do the same. Just keep in mind that the "Do as I say, not as I do" factor may come into play, so, when in doubt, just ask.

BE A TRAILBLAZER

You should always keep a basic blazer in your office or in your car—just in case. A blazer has the ability to make almost anything look work-ready—even a pair of jeans and a T-shirt—and it's an essential part of dressing for work in case of an unexpected meeting.

The blazer is interchangeable with your fitted girly jackets, three-quarter-length coats, and boxy jackets. Just make sure you are not confusing this necessity with outerwear.

These jackets can always bring any look up a notch or two.

CHAPTER 7

RSVP

EVENING AND EVENT DRESSING

$I\ can't\ think$ of any social situation more stressful to a woman than having to get glitzed up for a special event. There's the dress . . . and the shoes . . . and the jewelry . . . and the bag . . . and, oh my God, the underwear! Never mind the hair and makeup! Pretty soon, your brain goes reeling off in a thousand directions: "I should have lost ten pounds. I should have gotten a boob job. I should be five inches taller. Forget it—I'm not going."

Relax. And read this chapter.

I'm here to remind you that an evening out is not just a special event —it's a *style* event. It takes time and energy to prepare for it, because every component falls into the "different-from-everyday" category: the clothing, the accessories, and *you*. **You want to look sensational— and you want to feel extraordinary—and there are lots of tools out there to help you do it.**

Finding a dress is much easier if you approach the task with an open mind. When you have a strong mental picture and you try to match it, you'll never find what you want. Apparently, it just puts too much pressure on the shopping gods. So let go of the "ideal" concept, shift into flexible mode, and get out there and look around. The stores are filled with spectacular dresses, and one of them might even be the perfect one for you.

Sure, it's an effort. It's an effort for everyone. Even the celebrities you see in magazines have dozens of bells and whistles lurking underneath their twenty-thousand-dollar gowns. I cannot remember a woman I have successfully dressed for a special event who was not pushed up, corseted, girdled, seamless-pantied, Topsticked, duct-taped, jelly-boobed, or sewn into her seemingly perfect evening dress. If you have not experienced the pains and pleasures that go along with this style of dressing, you have not truly experienced evening wear to its fullest. This is the reality of the "real" woman.

It's time to accept the fact that preparing for a big event is not your everyday shopping trip. In fact, it can rank right up there with the adventure of a lifetime. So take a deep breath, gear up, and get ready for a gala journey.

Dresses

For the most part, you'll be looking at dresses that range from mid-calf to floor-length. There are some exceptions for formal daytime events, but cocktail dresses and gowns are the order of the evening.

A cocktail dress is the shorter of the two, and can run anywhere from a few inches below the knee to the ankle. A gown extends all the way to the floor, allowing for a sweeping entrance into a room. Some styles are longer still, pooling or trailing at the bottom. A long gown is extremely dressy and full of dramatic impact, making it the perfect choice for a very formal evening. It is appropriate when an event is deemed black-tie, or when your invitation includes the words "premiere," "awards," "gala," "star-studded," "red carpet," or "ball." Otherwise, it's cocktail time.

Your body type will dictate the style of evening dress that's best for you. Paying particular attention to the three critical areas of your body—top, waistline, and bottom—look for dresses that feature elements to flatter each. Use the following guide to help get you started.

TOPS	BEST FOR . . .
Halter—Ties behind the neck, open through the chest, bares the shoulders	All body types, as long as you have good arms
Plunging—A deep V that shows a lot of cleavage, with sleeves, tank straps, or straps that cut high on the shoulder	All body types, depending on the style of sleeve or strap
Scoop neck—A wide, U-shaped neckline that bares the chest, with sleeves or straps	Pear, willow, apple, diamond, and half-pint; narrow shoulders and fuller busts
Spaghetti strap—Thick or thin straps that attach to the bodice with a sweetheart or straight neckline	All body types with good shoulders and arms
Square neck—An open neckline shaped like a half square, usually with a sleeve that is long, short, or capped, or a thicker tank strap	Pear, willow, half-pint; narrow shoulders and smaller busts
Strapless—A horizontal or sweetheart bustline without straps or sleeves	All body types with good shoulders and arms
Sweetheart—An open neckline shaped like the top of a heart, with straps or sleeves	All body types

WAISTLINES	BEST FOR . . .
Corset—A fitted bodice with a dropped V- or U-shaped waist, usually with boning or seaming details and support under the bust	Pear, willow, hourglass, rectangle; short-waisted women
Empire—A raised waistline that usually sits just below the bust, fitted or loose to the waist	Pear, willow, rectangle, half-pint; smaller and fuller busts, depending on the bodice
Ruched—Pleats and gathers in the fabric at the waistline, forming an X or a V, or wrapped around the entire bodice below the bust to the waist	Hourglass, apple, rectangle, half-pint; no-waisters and fuller tummies
Sash—A tight, wide tie from the top of the waist to the hip	Willow, hourglass, rectangle; no-waisters
Sunburst—A shirring of fabric that resembles a sunburst, starting with a small point at one side of the waist and opening up across the bodice	Hourglass, apple, rectangle, half-pint; no-waisters and fuller tummies
Wrap—A crisscross of fabric that defines the waist and bust and fuller tummies	Willow, hourglass, apple, rectangle, half-pint; no-waisters

BOTTOMS	BEST FOR . . .
A-line—A skirt that flares gently from the hip down	All body types
Full—A skirt with volume underneath that stops at the knee or falls to the floor	Willow, hourglass, diamond, rectangle; half-pint in shorter skirts only
Handkerchief—A hemline of varying lengths falling in gentle asymmetrical points or flutes	All body types
Mermaid—Fitted through the waist and hips, with a flare at the knee or below	Willow, hourglass, diamond, rectangle, half-pint
Pleated—Multiple pleats or folds in the skirt from the waist down—vertical, horizontal, or forming a pattern—reaching anywhere from the knee to the floor; A-line or fitted	Apple and diamond in an A-line, hourglass in fitted, willow in both, half-pint in both to the knee
Ruffled—Fabric gathered into a frill, with a seam or piping along the edge for weight	Diamond, hourglass, willow, rectangle, half-pint
Straight—Narrow like a column, reaching to the knee or floor	Willow, hourglass, apple, diamond; half-pint in knee length
Tiered—A multi-layered skirt bottom, with separate horizontal or asymmetrical panels that fall in tiers upon each other	Willow, hourglass, rectangle, diamond
Waterfall—A hemline that is shorter in the front and longer in the back, baring the legs at the knee or ankle, and sometimes reaching to the floor	All body types

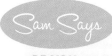

BE YOU

Don't ever try to copy a celebrity's look exactly. You can't decide that you want to be Jennifer Aniston at your ten-year reunion, and take off on a quest for the dress she wore when she won her Emmy. This is not about being Jennifer Aniston. It's about you loving the color or style of Jen's dress, knowing that what flatters you may be different from what flatters her, and using this knowledge as inspiration for *your* dress. Your goal is to look and feel like the ultimate version of yourself, not someone else. Your personality and the style of the dress must be in harmony to make it all work.

The casual shopper always stumbles upon a find when she least expects it, especially with evening wear. And that's when you know the dress is a wow—when it actually finds you.

Think of your prom dress or your wedding dress. When you put it on, you just knew it was perfect . . . or at least I hope you did. The room went silent, there was magic in the air, and all things pointed to the fact that this was *the* dress.

That's the same feeling you should get from a special-occasion dress. When you look in the mirror and "Wow!" is the first thing that comes to your mind, it's a true indicator that this is the dress for you. It's wow or nothing when it comes to event dressing.

Separates

Separates are always a wonderful option in the evening, as long as they're special enough to go the distance. One of the pieces should be glamorous and strong with some noticeable detail, while the other should be solid and simpler for balance. It could be as easy as a beaded skirt and a simple cashmere T-shirt, or a fantastic printed silk blouse with a dressy dark pant. Sometimes both pieces can be in the same fabric, creating a dresslike silhouette. As long as you don't overwhelm yourself with pattern, you'll be fine.

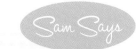

Formal Suits

An evening suit or lady's tuxedo can add glamour to your night on the town. Look for suiting in a more formal fabric, perhaps one that has a sheen or some Lurex pinstripes—metallic threads—running through it to add sparkle and sophistication. If you don't want to spend a lot of money, try wearing a formal top under a basic black suit. A lace, beaded, or sequined tank or camisole will make it evening-ready.

A lady's tuxedo makes a strong, sexy, decidedly stylish statement for a night out, and can be worn in a lighter shade for a daytime event. The style of your tux can be double-breasted for drama (always keep it buttoned, please) or single-breasted for simplicity. Select basic black, champagne, or any neutral color, and look for piping in a contrasting fabric.

To punctuate your tuxedo look, go for details that make it feminine, such as an exaggerated lapel or studded buttons. Try wearing it without a top underneath. Just be sure to accessorize it with a collar or choker necklace or strong earrings, so your chest area does not appear too bare. Never wear an evening suit with a visible bra as your underpinning. Even if the bra is gorgeous and cost a hundred bucks, it still comes across as tasteless and inappropriate.

Evening Fabrics—Fabulous, Forgiving

An evening dress is defined by certain details and design elements—an exquisite embellishment, a well-placed ruffle, a waterfall hemline, a fuller skirt, a single bared shoulder. But the primary feature that sets an evening dress apart from an everyday dress is fabric—beautiful, dramatic, sensual fabric.

It may have a sheen that catches the light in a certain way. It may be flowing and romantic. It may be very ornate, allowing you to sparkle your way into the night. The fabric tells you immediately that these are special dresses meant for something out of the ordinary.

Satin is a striking fabric for an evening dress. Usually made from silk or rayon, it comes in either a glossy or a matte finish. Satin has a sophistication that can glamorize even the most basic styles, and is easy for most body types to wear. A dense weave can hide most flaws with ease, but thinner satins have a tendency to cling to trouble spots. So choose structure as often as possible in a fabric like this.

Most silk is lightweight and sheer, with a lovely movement and flow. It is impeccable in a romantic style of dress, such as an empire waist or a slip dress. It has the least amount of structure of all the evening fabrics, which means you'd better have the body—or at least the undergarments—to back it up.

Lace is conservative and sweet, but can also be provocative in the right cut of dress. You can opt for proper in a style that is not too revealing, such as an A-line to the knee. Or you can kick things up a notch with a lacy style that is sinful and flirtatious: a low-plunging evening gown or a youthful cocktail minidress.

Matte jersey is a popular fabric for an evening dress. It is a flat-knit fabric that can have a bit of give and stretch without having Lycra in its makeup. When jersey is doubled—meaning

COLOR MAKES AN IMPACT

When determining a color for an evening dress, start with shades that make your eyes stand out, that set off your skin tone, and that flatter your hair color. Also choose a color that is right for the season.

Summer colors are bright and vivid. Choose pink, tangerine, lemon yellow, turquoise, lime green, and violet. Winter colors are generally deep jewel tones, such as ruby red, citrine orange, amethyst purple, sapphire blue, smoky topaz brown, and emerald green. The spring palette is clean and pale, with shades like soft pink, sherbet orange, butter yellow, grass green, sky blue, and lilac purple. Autumn colors are rich and warm, and include berry red, pumpkin orange, yellow ocher, espresso brown, avocado green, teal blue, and eggplant purple. When in doubt, black can serve you well for all occasions.

White evening dresses are acceptable only in the summer months. In the cooler months, it's all about winter whites, which have a soft gray or creamy tone. Make sure the style of your white dress is nowhere near the wedding variety. To be safe, choose a cocktail length.

Q I can hardly ever find a dress off the rack that fits right without tailoring. What are my options when it comes to a custom-made dress? Are they really expensive?

A Sometimes having a dress made for you is cheaper than spending tons of time shopping—not to mention tons of money on undergarments and visits to your tailor. Shop around, because there are plenty of good seamstresses and tailors who will charge a reasonable price to make something that is perfectly fitted to your body.

My advice is to stay involved with the process. Make sure you help select the fabric and style that will do you justice. Have several fittings and a trial run in a muslin version so you can see where it's all going. Talk specifically about the timeframe and the price. A 50 percent deposit is usually required, and you should pay the balance only when the dress is completed and you are happy with the results. Always make sure you take your foundation garments and heels with you to every fitting, since they can change everything.

two layers of fabric make up the dress—it can have wonderful body and be very structured. When it's not doubled, watch out, because it will hug everything in sight.

Crepe is usually found in silk or polyester, and is both light and sturdy, with a slightly crinkled texture. It is one of my favorite fabrics, because it's thin and light, yet has enough control to hold its shape well. Stunning in a spaghetti-strap cocktail dress or a long, dramatic gown, it hugs the right curves and gives you freedom of movement throughout the night.

Sequins, beading, and embroidery add brilliant life to any fabric, and are the novelty choices when you want your dress to sparkle and shine. These embellishments can enhance and complement almost any fabric, such as satin, silk, and lace. A short sequined cocktail dress, a beaded lace gown, and an embroidered satin strapless will all speak for themselves at any event. If you opt for a style with this sort of detail, be prepared to stand out. Remember that the dress is now the accessory, so tone down every other element of your look to the minimum. Too much of a good thing is still too much.

In some cases, the dress you select may be available in a combination of fabrics. That's what makes it interesting and "evening." Look for details, seaming, and cuts that flatter your body's unique shape and curve, and fabrics that forgive the flaws. Start with styles you love to wear every day, and experiment from there.

Pouring Your Own Foundation

After everything I've just said, you might get the impression that style, fit, fabric, and color are the most important elements to consider when buying an event dress. But, believe it or not, they're actually the *second*-most-important considerations. The items that rise to number one on the event-dressing checklist? The undergarments.

A great dress is nothing without a great foundation. And this is where my bag of tricks is about to spill wide open, so pay close attention as we explore what goes on behind the velvet ropes of the best event dresses.

We'll start with the most basic undergarment, the bra. You want one that gives you the best amount of lift and separation, while working with the style of dress you have selected. If cleavage is a must, then so is a padded push-up bra. If the dress has a plunging neckline, a low-cut or demi bra is necessary.

If you're wearing a halter-style or low-back dress, you must have a convertible bra that can handle the dress's

RSVP

A dress code on your invitation is a great indicator of exactly what you should be wearing to a specific event and should always be followed out of respect for your host. Use these guidelines when a dress code is stipulated for your next RSVP, and you'll be properly dressed.

COCKTAIL

Any length of dress is fine as long as it is elegant. However, a floor-length dress may seem a bit over-the-top unless it's the dead of winter. Opt for a shorter, "cocktail" style as often as possible, or a fabulous skirt-and-top ensemble.

BLACK TIE

A long gown, a dressy evening separate, and a knee-length cocktail dress are appropriate— nothing shorter. Always have a wrap on hand to cover your shoulders, at least upon arrival.

WHITE TIE

This is the ultimate in formal dressing. A long gown is a must, paired with a long white glove, which you will remove for dinner and replace for dancing. A wrap is always a good idea for this extremely formal affair.

real style secret

THE TWIST

One of my favorite secrets for getting some extra cleavage out of the basic bra is to try "the twist." Twist the bra around one or two times at the center that connects the two cups. It becomes tighter, pulling your breasts together for extra lift and cleavage. It's a breast enhancement in seconds flat.

THE NEXT-BEST THING

If the dress you choose for your special event will not accommodate a bra but you truly need one, have the next-best thing sewn into your dress. Your tailor can tack two foam pads to the inside of the bodice or within the lining, giving you support, lift, and extra cleavage. You must be wearing the dress and standing in front of a mirror when this alteration is done, so you can decide on the placement of the pads to achieve the right balance. The total cost? Less than the price of a good bra on sale—around fifteen bucks.

THE SURGICAL-TAPE ALTERNATIVE

Though I love what duct tape can do for breast enhancements, there *is* a less painful solution. I have found that stretchy, clear surgical tape is just as effective as duct tape—if not more so. It gives excellent support, it's easier to work with and remove, and the stretch factor allows you to use less of it. In case you run into trouble along the way, have a close friend on hand to help you get to those hard-to-reach spots—at least the first time. Grab a roll of surgical tape on your next visit to the drugstore and give it a try.

special needs. Under no circumstances should you allow your bra straps—or any other part of your bra—to show. If there is no way to wear a regular bra with your dress, you have your choice of stick-on bras, stick-on jelly boobs, or even duct tape.

Yes, you read that correctly—duct tape. This age-old tradition of building up the breast probably got its start in the pageant circuit. It is sometimes the only solution in television, film, and print fashion emergencies, because the tape is invariably lying around somewhere. I've learned to make an A cup look like a C, but it takes some experimentation and practice.

The idea is to lift the breast up and press the tape in place, creating an L around it that supports the breast from underneath and pushes it in from the side to create cleavage. It may take a few strips of tape to get the right amount of lift, depending on the size of your bust. Although it can be a bit uncomfortable, it really works. You can remove the tape at the end of the night with some vitamin E oil or body lotion. Use this technique as a worst-case-scenario option, and try it out well in advance of the event.

There are many other options for creating cleavage and fullness, and, to tell you the truth, I'm not especially fond of most of them. Though jelly inserts—or "chicken cutlets," as I call them—are wonderful in theory, they are not the most effective choice. They are tucked into a bra to fill it out and give it shape, but they are heavy, sometimes dragging the bust down instead of lifting it up. And I am told that they are too warm, causing the wearer to sweat, which is never fashionable.

A stick-on jelly bra is much the same. This is a flesh-colored jelly molded into the shape of a breast, with a washable, reusable adhesive backing that sticks onto the breast and clips together in the front with a clear closure. Unfortunately, jelly bras barely hold anything up, and I've found they work only on A and B cups. Aside from giving a smooth shape and hiding the nipple, this novelty is not good for much.

The peel-and-stick fabrics that act as a bra are made of a thin, paperlike material shaped like the cup of a bra and backed with adhesive. In my experience, their effectiveness is limited to smaller breasts. They are often hard to apply, and because they never seem to lie smoothly, they can sometimes be detected under a thin dress. Give them a shot if you like. You may be one of the lucky ones for whom they work like a charm.

IT'S GOTTA GO SOMEWHERE

When you wear foundation garments, the extra fat, skin, and chubbiness you're trying to control and conceal do not disappear entirely. Pity. It's gotta go somewhere, and sometimes it's up and over, and sometimes it's down and out. The excess can spill over the top of your corset, around your bust, under your arms, and over your back. Sometimes, it can creep down from under the seams of your girdle, pooling around your thighs.

If any of this occurs, try going up a size in the slimmer. With a corset, adjust the hook and eye to loosen things up a bit. An effective trick is to lean forward and drop all the excess into the cup of your bra or corset— no bulge, and more boob to boot.

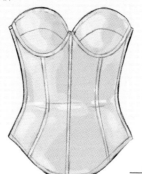

I've saved my most trusted solution for last—simple latex-foam padded inserts. They are lightweight, comfortable, and easy to use. Place them in a basic padded or unpadded bra for excellent enhancement, underneath the breast for lift, and on the side of the breast for cleavage. You can find these enhancers at fabric stores or on pageant Web sites. Do an Internet search and order by cup size.

Always remember that wearing a bra and having a good amount of support and lift will make your tummy seem flatter and your torso appear longer. That's because you are increasing the distance between the bottom of your breast and your stomach, giving the illusion of length. When the bra is not doing enough of the lifting for you, it's time to get serious. Introducing . . . the corset.

The corset is extraordinary for event dressing, and is a must if you don't have time to slim down naturally before a special event. The best ones will cost a bit more, because they're made the old-fashioned way, with heavy satin and boning. But the amount of structure you get—the lift, support, and tummy control—is second to none.

Quality corseting can be miraculous when it comes to shrinking the waistline. In fact, I have taken a woman from a size 6 to a size 2 using a corset-and-slimmer combination, whittling almost six inches off her waist.

It is essential to decide if you will be wearing a corset before you finalize the selection of your event dress. Since a good corset can take you down almost two sizes, you'll need to know where you're going to land on the size chart before

THE MAGIC OF TOPSTICK

Here's one secret that could have gone in every chapter of this book, and I have to say it's one of my best and most indispensable tricks of the trade. Topstick is clear, double-sided medical tape that was designed originally to hold a wig in place. That all changed when Jennifer Lopez wore her famous green dress to the Grammy Awards one year and defied gravity. I was there, and even I was in awe.

Now the secret is out. This stuff works so well that I carry a box of it in my styling kit, one in my bag, and one in the car—just in case. It is a staple in event dressing and a plus in everyday dressing, making quick work of a falling hemline or a broken zipper. Try it when you want to hide a bra strap under a tank top, stick your dress to your undergarments to avoid a peep show, or keep your breasts from popping out when you wear a revealing dress or suit. Get addicted to the magic by visiting www.vapon.com.

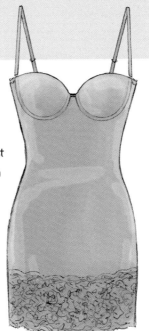

committing. It's best to put the dress you love on hold and then try it on with the corset for the proper size and fit.

For extra measure, combine the corset or your best bra option with a body slimmer or girdle. A slimmer can even out bumps and bulges while minimizing the tummy, back rolls, hips, and thighs. Because it is made of a slick, stretchy fabric that prevents clinging, it serves as an excellent foundation for a dress, allowing it to lie smooth for a beautiful, body-enhancing finish. Find one that is strong enough for control, but still comfortable enough to wear through the evening.

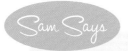
Once you've completed your choices in undergarments, it's smart to do a trial run and make sure everything is in place—and stays there. You can find undergarments that make you look and feel like a million, but if you can't sit down comfortably or bend over without spilling out or popping something, it doesn't matter how superb you look when you're standing still for photos. Form and function *must* be in harmony.

A night or two before the event, try it all on—including shoes and jewels—to make sure your ensemble allows you to do all the things you need to do with comfort and grace. That means sitting and standing, breathing normally, and even doing a little dance around the room.

Keep everything on for at least a half-hour, and if it all feels right and stays in place, you're fine. If there are any problems, you can address them well in advance of the big night. Event dressing is something like a performance, and you'll be happier when the dry run goes off without a hitch.

Now that you understand the best way to select your evening gear and what to wear underneath it, you have to pull together all the remaining elements. This leads us to the shoes, jewelry, bag, and wrap.

The Allure of the Shoe

An evening dress is outstanding with a high heel, because everything changes for the better when you boost your height. Your weight is distributed, and your posture shifts into place so you look slimmer. The additional few inches alter the way the dress falls on your body, making for a better fit. And a heel will visually correct—in a snap—a lot of proportion issues.

Even when you're just shopping for a dress, you should always try it on with a heel. Bring a pair with you, or ask your salesperson if there is a pair on hand for you to use—chances are, there will be.

If you must wear a lower heel or a flat, make sure it complements the dress and has a "special" quality to make it work for evening. A kitten heel is a good compromise, because, although it looks like a high heel from the front, it's actually closer to a flat. It's perfect for taller women who don't want to impose their height on their dates or tower over the room.

The front of the shoe is where the deception takes place. Whether you choose a kitten heel or a flat, make sure it has a pointed toe or some embellishment to distract from the lack of heel.

Of course, your shoes must coordinate with your dress, so make your choice based on both color and fabric. Upgrade the fabric to something dressy like satin or silk to match the mood of an evening dress. If your frock is simple, go to town with a shoe that stands out via color, style, or detail. If your dress is outrageous, tone down the shoe for balance.

When you can't find the shoe to match the dress, consider metallic leathers. Navy looks best with pewter, which is a darker twist on silver. Warm tones such as pinks, corals, oranges, and creams look best with gold, bronze, or copper, as do lighter shades of green. Cool colors such as purples, blues, grays, and true whites shine with silver. And black looks best with black, though you can also try playing with fun colors or variations of prints, patterns, and textures. Nude shoes are a last resort for hard-to-match evening wear, and should be reserved for summer.

Judicious Jewels

Evening and event jewelry should be more elaborate and special than your every-day basics. Diamonds, rhinestones, and colorful gems come into play, but you should make sure that they don't compete with your ensemble.

The stores are filled with specialty jewelry, and it's fun to shop for different pieces for your event. But please consider the big picture. Getting dressed up includes a lot of elements, and you don't want to risk looking like a Christmas tree.

So here's my tip for event jewelry. Excluding pins, which can go just about any-where, there are four major places where a woman can adorn herself with some cool jewels: ears, neck, wrist, and hand. I think earrings are fundamental for event dressing, so start there and choose two other areas of focus. Bottom line: It's either about earrings, a bracelet, and a ring, or earrings, a necklace, and a ring. You get the idea.

I love the simplicity of a beautiful earring, a few pretty bracelets layered on one wrist, and a ring on the opposing hand. Another favorite option is a deli-cate stud earring with a strong necklace and a simple cocktail ring. Mix it up and balance it out.

Remember, it's likely you're not Elizabeth Taylor, the walking diamond mine, able to pull off scads of jewels at one time. So stay within your comfort zone or maybe just a whisper outside it, and you'll be accessorized to perfection.

The Complementary Evening Bag

An evening bag should reflect and/or complement your dress in both fabric and color. When you're decked out in a fabulous dress, your bag should be an invisible accessory, so your outfit remains center stage. A simple silk or satin purse that matches your dress—and virtually disappears—is a good choice. Fortunately, these fabrics are dyeable, so getting the right shade is relatively easy.

If your dress is understated with clean, simple lines, your bag can be as bold as the Krupp Diamond. Go for broke with beads or sequins, vivid colors or metallics, embroidery or patterns.

In all instances, keep an evening bag relatively small, and *never* overstuff it or you'll ruin its lines. You don't need to carry much anyway: a few dollars, keys, ID, lipstick, a compact, and some mints. Your bag should also balance the size of your frame. If you're a larger woman, a teeny bag will look like it was meant for a little girl. Use what you've learned in Chapter 2 to keep proportion in sync.

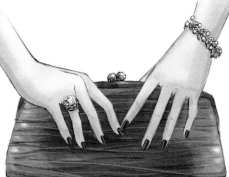

It's a Wrap

The real finishing touch in evening and event dressing is the cover-up. What will it be, ladies? A wrap or a shawl? A shrug or a fur stole? A long or short evening jacket? I'll describe, you decide!

Wraps and shawls are always wonderful. The fabric of your dress will dictate your choice, and the weather will dictate the weight. As a rule, wraps and shawls work well over any dress, long or short, that does not have a sleeve—strapless, spaghetti strap, tank, shift, and the like.

If your dress is basic black, an ornate wrap is in order. If you are sparkling and glitzy, choose a solid. If you're wearing a pattern or print, go for a base color that is predominant in your dress. In the winter, your best fabric

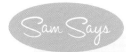

THE PASHMINA BACKLASH IS OVER

The pashmina was a huge trend a few years back that took the fashion industry by storm. These expensive wraps were seen everywhere—from formal dinner parties to the grocery store. Women were clamoring to collect them in every color, and why not? But then came the backlash.

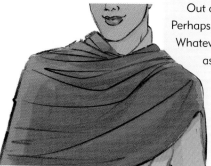

Out of nowhere, the pashmina became the butt of all jokes, a fashion don't. Perhaps it was because they were being knocked off in cheaper varieties. Whatever the reason, the drama has died down. The pashmina has resurfaced as a basic wrap, so feel free to wear one with reckless abandon.

Pashminas work for both day and night, and suit any style of dress— from strapless to tank to sleeved. Try a color that's either a shade lighter or darker than your dress, for some pop. If a little black dress is on the agenda, a boldly colorful pashmina in a wonderful jewel tone will impress.

choices are wool, cashmere, and pashmina, which is a luxurious one-ply wrap made of cashmere and silk. In summer, satins and silks are best.

A shrug is the novelty version of a wrap. Think of a shawl with sleeves that cover the shoulders and arms, and a body that ends just below the breast line. The shrug came into vogue in the thirties, and was commonly worn over an evening dress. The style keeps the dress in the limelight, giving you just a hint of coverage.

A fur stole or chubby (a jacketlike version of the shrug, with a longer bodice and three-quarter sleeves), either real or faux, is a stunning choice as a glamorous cover-up. Undeniably elegant, it is reserved exclusively for the cooler months. A fur stole can add that Old Hollywood vibe to a long, dramatic evening dress, and can lend a touch of urban cool to a cocktail dress.

Evening coats, whether long or short, are most often solid and simple, made in a heavy fabric with a soft sheen. They can also be brocade, busy and decorative, like an opera coat. They have very clean lines, usually with a bit of an A-line and a shorter sleeve that begs to be worn with a delicate glove. Their collars are mostly small or banded, so as not to complicate the look. Choose these jackets and coats according to the dress code of your event, because they tend to make a grand statement upon arrival.

Obviously, there are many elements to think about when you dress for a special event. At least a little effort is involved, but now you have the tools to add some dazzle to your evening without the stress.

CHAPTER 8

Behind the Seams

TAILORING

Behind every great woman is a great tailor. Learning to select the right clothing for your body type makes you sensible, but getting it to fit properly is an art form. Once you master this important style lesson and develop an eye for the ultimate fit, you'll unlock your potential to look your absolute best in whatever you wear. Part of having real style is knowing, at a glance, when an item of clothing can go one step further and be that much better. Wearing the "right clothes" is always secondary to having a meticulous fit, because, without it, even the most spectacular outfit fades into mediocrity.

Tailoring helps to elevate your wardrobe—both the basics and the special pieces—to the next level. Its purpose is to improve the fit of an item—not completely remake the basic style or cut.

I've talked a lot about proportion and how the right fit can correct almost any issue. Now I'll show you how to look at your clothing in a strategic way so you begin to see how the slightest change in a hem or seam can affect the big picture. By the end of this chapter, you'll be able to walk into a tailoring shop and know exactly what needs to be done to each piece of your clothing to make it outstanding. Once you understand the "how to" of altering your clothing correctly, you can work with your tailor to turn your store-bought clothing into couture.

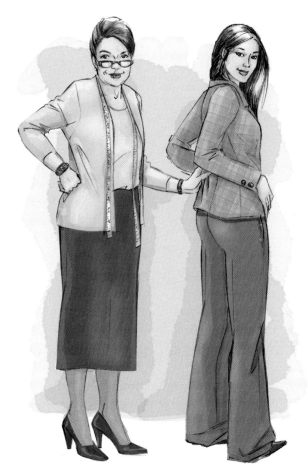

You and Your Tailor

When purchasing a new item of clothing that requires altering, ask your salesperson if tailoring is included. Most of the time, there is a fee to have the work done in-house, but some high-end specialty stores—and even chain stores that you would never suspect—offer their clients free alterations. A penny saved is a penny you can spend on something else, so always ask.

Based on your budget, you will need to decide the caliber of expert you are looking for. If you want a quick and inexpensive fix, try the tailor at your dry cleaner's. I am often surprised and impressed by the speed and quality of the work at these shops.

If you have an item that is more important to you, step up to a mid-range tailor or seamstress. Odds are you will be paying more, so you should also expect more precision and attention to detail.

Lastly, if you have a very special piece that you've spent some serious cash on, head straight to an exceptional tailor. Hold on to your hat, though, because prices at these shops can be astronomical. I have often turned beet red at the cash register when faced with the total cost of some of my alterations.

Try a little experimenting with the tailors in your area. Start with alterations on just one piece, and check out the results. Over time, you'll have your own little black book of qualified professionals in a variety of price ranges.

Whether you use the services of a lower-end or top-of-the-line tailor, always ask what the charge will be before you commission him or her to alter something for you. You're the one who ultimately decides if it's worth the price, so don't hesitate to change your mind if the cost seems too high. After all, if it's going to run you $450 to remake a three-year-old $500 leather jacket, it makes more sense to buy a new one.

A truly good tailor will be able to look at you and know exactly what must be done to an item of clothing to make you look your best. But I've learned over the years that tailoring should also be a team effort. You need to be involved in the process, and, more important, must be informed about the plan of action.

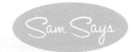

Sam Says

STOP OFF AND DROP OFF

When you're driving away from the mall with your new, needs-to-be-altered purchase on the seat beside you, don't head home just yet. Immediately drop it off at your tailor's. This is the best way to avoid the temptation of wearing something before it's just right. If the shop is closed or you don't have the time, leave the purchase in your car to remind you to take it in for a little surgery at your earliest convenience.

real style secret

LEARNING TO SPEAK "INCH"

Have you ever gone to the salon and asked to have your hair cut a few inches, indicating how much you mean by holding up your finger and thumb with the desired amount between them? Then you look in the mirror, expecting a certain length, but instead are shocked by your new bob?

The same kind of horror can apply when you drop off a skirt at the tailor, finger and thumb poised, with the simple instruction to "shorten the hem this much." You need to talk to your tailor in *inches*, because that's the language he or she understands. One inch or two can make a huge difference in the way something looks on you.

You're the one who looks in the mirror every day, so by now you should know your problem areas. In fact, I'm sure you know them by heart. The best thing about tailors is that they look at you in a different way, much as a stylist would, with a fresh perspective and an objective eye. They may be able to correct flaws you've never even noticed, or can work with you to solve age-old problems you thought could never be fixed. Teamwork is the name of the game, and it will allow you to reap the benefits of this great relationship.

You'll need to start by knowing what can and should be tailored, and why. We'll begin at the bottom and work our way up.

Perfecting Your Pants

The most common alteration is done on the hem of a pant, skirt, or dress. In most cases the hem is being shortened, but for those of you with longer legs, some lengthening may be in order. Either way, this is probably the easiest and most inexpensive way to polish the look of your favorite bottoms.

Let's look at pants first. Determining the length of your pants is a very personal thing. Your preference comes into play here, but the right length also hinges on the length of your legs, the height of the shoe you'll be wearing, and any proportion issues you may need to correct.

The longer the hem, the longer your leg line appears. Remember, the general rule is to have the bottom hem of your pants stop three-quarters of an inch above the bottom of the heel of your shoe when you're standing.

Certain looks, like boot-cut pants paired with a heel, demand a longer length. Capris worn with flats can be significantly shorter. When in doubt, ask. Your tailor can help you make the right decision.

Always take along at least two pairs of shoes in varying heights and styles to make sure your pant length is correct. If the pants are for a special occasion, bring the shoes you will be wearing to the event, to guarantee the perfect length.

You must determine whether or not you prefer a "break" in the hem of your pants. (A break is like an interruption in the line of your pants, causing a "dent" at the ankle and allowing a bit of extra fabric to fall below it.) Too much break can make your pants look sloppy—not enough, and it's floodsville. To complicate things further, the height of your heel will change the break considerably. So, when you find a length you like, try it with varying heels, and check the hemline from both the front and the back.

Tapering is another kind of alteration done to make an item leaner and create more shape or curve. It can be done only along the seam of a garment. In most cases, tapering is done on a gradient—with the amount of fabric taken in getting progressively smaller—but it can also be done in a straight line.

You can actually taper your bottoms to flatter your figure. Tapering from the knee down will remove some flare and make the leg straighter. You can taper a fuller leg from just below the seat to the knee, streamlining the thigh area to make your legs appear longer and leaner. Taper this area when the shape of your thighs gets lost behind the fullness of the fabric, or when the line of your pants looks too straight. This can be done along the outside seam or the inseam.

The above solution works only with boot-cut pants, because their wider flare serves as a contrast to your leaner-looking thighs. But be cautious. If your hips and thighs are very full, this kind of tapering will have the reverse effect, making

ONE PIN OR TWO?

When altering your pant length, the tailor may use only one pin as a marker in the back of the leg. This means that the hem will be straight across when finished—the same length in the front as in the back. When the pant is double-pinned, in the front and the back, chances are the hemline will be on a slight angle and a bit longer in the back than the front to accommodate a heel. Always ask what you're getting, so there are no surprises after the fact. Personally, I prefer two pins, so the hem is shorter in the front to prevent excess bunching.

MOVE IT OR LOSE IT

What if you've gained a few pounds, and your favorite pants are tight around your middle and don't have seam allowances in the waist? If you're not ready to lose the pants just yet, there's an easy solution. Simply cut off the button, move it over on the waistband to give you a tad more room, and sew it back on, and you'll gain about three-quarters of an inch. Just be sure that the button will reach its hole before you reattach it, and the zipper still zips properly. With a few simple pulls of the needle and thread, you're your own master tailor and you've rescued your pants from the giveaway pile.

those areas look larger by comparison. In such cases, it's better for you to keep the straight line intact.

In all instances, tapering in the leg should be kept to a minimum. If you have to do too much, you're probably buying the wrong size or style.

If you are one of the millions of women who walk around with a gaping space in the back of the waistband on your pants or jeans, let a tailor help. The waistband can always be taken in or tapered for the right fit. It can even be removed completely and reattached lower on your hips to drop the waistline. (This complicated alteration is best left to a very skilled tailor.)

Normally, when you take in the waistband of your pants, the seat must follow. If not, the result will be a tighter waistband and a larger, sloppier butt below it. This simple alteration is done by making a gradual V-shaped taper in the yoke on the back of your pants. You can also take the seat in along the back center seam if there is too much fabric bunching over your rear.

When you're not taking things in or up, you're letting them out. This is usually the last thing any of us wants to do, unless you're tall and need the extra length in your hemline. For the rest of us, letting clothing out means we've gained an inch or two somewhere along the way, and we're in dire need of more breathing room.

Here's where tailoring can actually save you some money. Instead of buying something new, find out if there is enough seam allowance to let out your favorite pants or skirt so you can wear them or it without turning blue.

Seam allowances are usually found on pants or skirts, although sometimes you'll get lucky with a dress, jacket, or shirt. To locate seam allowances, turn the

real style secret

CUPPING

I learned this alteration from a dear celebrity friend while getting her ready for the Oscars. Cupping is the best way to get some serious shape and curve in the booty area. Here's how it's done.

Beginning below the bottom of the butt, the center seam is tapered slightly to the back of the knee. The curve of the butt is "cupped" by the fabric, creating the slightest lift. When you stand in profile, the fabric hugs your backside instead of draping over it.

I still find it amazing that one simple alteration can generate such a body-enhancing benefit. This is definitely one of Hollywood's best-kept style secrets that you should try for yourself.

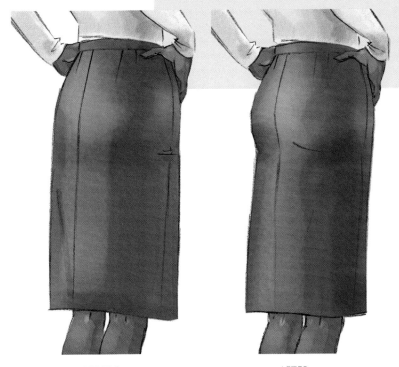

BEFORE   AFTER

LONGER LEGS CAN GO THE DISTANCE

If you're a leggy girl, always look for pants that have seam allowance in the hem. Even if the length is right when you buy them, it's a good idea to have some extra fabric to allow for shrinkage. Most pants will have at least two inches of extra fabric that is turned under at the hem. Even if you don't see it, chances are it's there.

If the pants are too short but the seam allowance is there, take them to a tailor—tags on —and have the hem let out, pressed, and pinned to the proper length. If they're still too short, have your tailor return the hem to its original state, take the pants back to the store, and try, try again.

garment inside out and check to see if extra fabric is folded back and pressed flat around the seams. The presence of this fabric will allow your tailor to open the garment and increase its size.

Normally, you can get almost an inch extra on side seams, and a maximum of two inches in the waist and seat. That's not bad, really, considering that most of us grow and shrink about that much during the year. When things get tight, let 'em all out. It's a much better solution to keep you looking good and eliminating the overhang around your waist.

The final alterations you can do on your pants have to do with front pockets and the rise of your pants. Though pockets may be functional, they are rarely flattering, especially if you carry any extra weight in your hips and thighs. Unless you have no hips and need the pockets for balance to fill you out, I say get rid of them. How many pants have you tried on that would have been flawless if it weren't for those darn pockets?

Talk to your tailor about options, because the pocket style will dictate the alteration. First, you can have the pockets closed and sewn down—stitched on the outside seam in a matching thread. You may leave them inside in case you change your mind, but odds are you won't. Once you see how much smoother your pants lie on your hips and thighs, you'll want 'em out for good.

When you reach this conclusion, you'll want to take advantage of option number two for all future pocket alterations: cutting them out. This alteration works on any type of pocket, but it's best when the pocket is a vertical slash located exactly on the side seam of your pants or skirt. The pocket can be removed in its entirety. The hem is closed as if it were the side seam to begin with. The look?

THREE SEAMS THE CHARM

When you decide to alter the waist and seat of your pants, you may introduce some new issues. Many pants and even skirts have some sort of pocketing in the back, and taking in the center seam will inevitably bring the two pockets closer together. This is a huge no-no. The solution? Have your tailor split the difference between the center seam and the two side seams. A little bit is taken in from all three areas, keeping the pockets in the right place but still getting the job done. The result is the fit you're looking for without compromising the garment's style.

Like the pocket never existed at all. Ask your tailor if your pants are eligible for this alteration.

Last but not least, the rise of your pants can be altered. Remember, this area runs along the length of your zipper or button fly to the crotch. Sometimes there can be one or two inches of extra fabric at the end of the fly, which can make the pant look as if it were made for a man rather than a woman. Shortening the rise removes the extra fabric from the crotch area and corrects the problem.

This is not my favorite alteration. It's a tricky one to do, and it can be a real hassle, because it never seems to turn out quite right. If the pants fit poorly in the rise, reconsider purchasing them. But if you insist, find an expert tailor to get the job done properly.

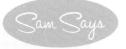

WHITE PANTS? POCKETS OUT!

Why oh why do manufacturers of white pants even bother putting pockets in them? Can't they just add fake pockets for show and detail? There is nothing cute about white pants with a clump of pocketing showing through. Most of the time, it ends up looking like rumpled underwear. Is this some sort of inside joke? Please always have the pockets on your white pants removed. Front and back. Stat. Thank you.

Altering Skirts and Dresses

There's probably not a woman alive who hasn't had this experience: You're standing in front of the mirror in the fitting room, trying on a dress or skirt. You love the style, the color, the cut, and the fabric, but something is a little off. You turn this way and that, trying to figure it out, and it finally hits you. The length is too long, and it's taking you from potentially fabulous to borderline frumpy.

Well, don't give up that great find just yet, because raising the hemline can make a world of difference in the way dresses and skirts look on your body. Introducing the second-most-common alteration for women.

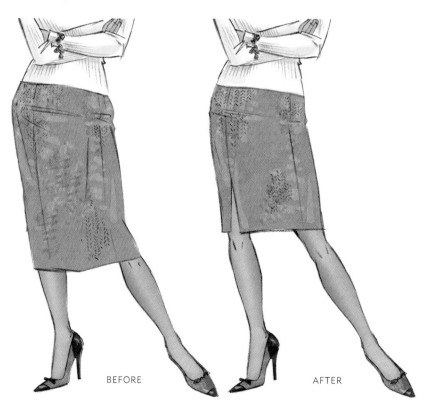

BEFORE   AFTER

The way you feel about your legs will determine the final length of your skirts and dresses. Of course, the right heel comes into play, as well. If you have gorgeous legs from ankle to high thigh, you can get away with just about any length. But if you're like most women, there's a point on your leg where it goes from good to not so good. And that's the spot you want to pay attention to.

If your legs lose their sex appeal just above the knee, then a length that's to the knee or just below it is best for you. If you're great to mid-thigh, you can go shorter. Most women will find that they have at least two variations that do them justice.

On a skirt or dress, tapering is much the same as on a pant. The placement of the seam will determine where the tapering occurs. You can slightly taper the side seams on an A-line for a narrower fit, or go more extreme and turn it into a pencil style. The waist of a skirt can be taken in on the back center seam. On a dress, this alteration is usually done on the side seams to hug your curves and create more shape.

real style secret

WHEN THE DRESS SAYS NO

When shortening a dress or skirt, be sure that the length does not compromise the line of the garment. You may look terrific in a mini, but that doesn't mean everything you buy should be altered accordingly. Sometimes, the dress says no.

The designer will always give you a clue about the best length for a particular dress or skirt, and that's the length it is when you find it on the rack. So, to maximize its look—and yours—stay within a few inches of that guideline when tailoring. Don't fight the style too much by overaltering. You may ruin the proportions and throw the whole look off balance. Ask for your tailor's professional opinion, and work together to find the best length—for your body and for the dress.

Topping It All Off

Now let's move on to the upper half of your body. Alterations on tops and jackets can include the length, width, body, shoulder, and sleeve. And, as with your pants, these fixes will usually involve shortening, letting out, tapering, and a wonderful little thing called darting.

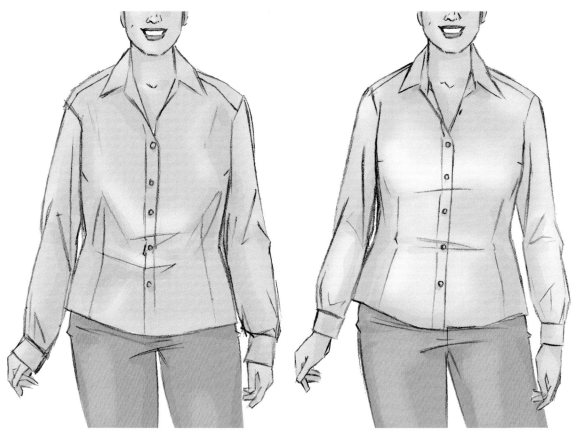

BEFORE   AFTER

A dart is a type of seam that *does not* join two panels of fabric together, but can be sewn anywhere on a garment to nip it in. The most common place for darting is under the bustline or below the shoulder blades on a dress, top, or jacket. Darts should always run parallel to each other, opposing each other for balance. They can run up and down or on an angle, hugging the waist or giving the illusion of one. They can also be featured diagonally on the sides of the breast to create structure and shape.

Use darts to reinvent your existing wardrobe. They can make fuller shirts more feminine, and can soften the lines of boxy jackets and outerwear. When the curve of your body gets lost behind the excess fabric on the front or back panel of a top, a dart can give you back some of your contours.

If you're that girl who stands in front of the mirror and pulls the excess fabric of your tops behind your back until you like what you see, if you've lost some weight or your clothes could use some refining, then it's time for tapering. Unlike a dart, tapering can be performed only along a seam that joins two panels. Tops can be tapered along the side seams, down the back center seam, or along the seam of a sleeve. Tapering gets rid of any bulk and allows the clothing to follow the lines of *your* body, not the stock body of the fit model used to make the garment.

Letting out the seams of shirts and jackets is a much less common alteration. Shirts and tops rarely have enough seam allowance, so if the bust or waist of your top is too tight and there's not enough fabric to let out, it's probably time to purchase a new one. Jackets, especially the suit variety, are more likely to have seam allowances. The back center seam, the side seams, and the sleeve may be released for additional length or more room.

The length of jackets and tops can be as crucial for your body proportions as pant length, yet very few women take advantage of this notion in tailoring. You can correct so many issues by shortening a top that you plan to wear untucked, especially if you are on the short side.

A Tailoring leather is an art, so it should be left to the best of the best. Sometimes that means an exceptional tailor, and other times, believe it or not, it means your shoe guy. Cobblers work with leather more frequently than most tailors do, so they have greater skill in this area. What's more, they are likely to have the machines and equipment to handle the job.

For example, tailoring leather often requires a special needle that is designed to pass easily through the thick hide. Often, your leather pieces must be glued instead of sewn, even if they are crazy expensive and from the best designer collections. On the other hand, it might surprise you to know that leather pants may be best shortened with a simple snip of the scissors, the hem left raw and unfinished. When you decide to have your leather tailored, be sure to ask what kind of work needs to be done and how it will be accomplished.

When shortening the length of a jacket, caution is critical to maintain proportions. Let's say you buy a blazer that's too long in the body, making you look shorter than you are. If the jacket does not have pockets at the waist, you may be able to have the bottom hem taken up a small amount. If it does have pockets, shortening from the bottom is probably out of the question.

Your best bet is to have it shortened by altering the jacket's horizontal seam, which runs across the top of the shoulders. Talk about costly! This is a major alteration, but it's the only way to get it truly right. If you choose to go this route, you'd better be absolutely sure you're in love with the jacket and prepared to spend whatever it takes.

Clearly, taking up the length of a jacket is a risky alteration. If it's not done correctly, the jacket can look like it's sawed off and way out of whack. So, even if the tailor says he can hem it from the bottom and it will look fine, think about my seventeen-hundred-dollar suit jacket that sits in my closet, ruined because it was shortened from the bottom instead of the shoulder. Then take another look at your options.

real style secret

After you have corrected the length of your tops and everything else is tapered or darted according to your womanly curves, you can turn your attention to the outskirts. These areas include the shoulders and sleeves.

Basically, the shoulder seam of your tops and jackets should stop where your shoulder ends. If your top has padded shoulders or additional structure, the seam may extend about half an inch beyond your shoulder and still be fine. Any more than that and it's tailor time.

Shoulder alterations can be costly, because they are time consuming. The sleeve must be detached to get the job done, and then reattached with care. Sometimes the shoulders can be brought together slightly by taking in the back center seam of a jacket all the way up through the collar or lapel. You can expect to pay a bit more in both of these situations, so these alterations should be done

Q **Can T-shirts be tailored effectively, or is it a silly idea?**

A I've always fantasized about going through my wardrobe, piling up all my T-shirts, and taking them in to be shortened. So I finally got off my butt and did just that. Well, I learned an important lesson for you.

Most T-shirt bottoms are stitched on a special factory machine that keeps them from getting stretched and pulled out of shape when they're sewn. Most tailors, however, do not have the same machines. So, though my newly shortened T-shirts were the right length, they had the shape of bell-bottom pants. Not cute. In the end, I searched until I found a T-shirt that balanced my proportions, and now I have thirty of them that I wear with pride.

Shortening the sleeves of your Ts can be much easier. Since there is less fabric to stretch, they generally turn out just fine.

only when absolutely necessary. For example, if you have an amazing designer top from the eighties with exaggerated shoulders that you are positive can be revived with a little help, then go for it.

Next on the alterations agenda is the sleeve length. Sometimes shortening a sleeve is necessary to rid you of sloppy, bunching arms. This is particularly important for a woman, because the grace of your limbs is among your best features, and you don't want to clutter it with excess fabric.

Most shirtsleeves can be tailored from the cuff and shortened according to your preference—whether you want to show more of your wrist or none at all. If you're unsure, ask your tailor for advice. For the most part, this is an inexpensive and common alteration.

When a suit-coat sleeve is altered, the sleeve is turned under and the decorative buttons that line the wrist are moved up accordingly. If the cuff or sleeve has a more elaborate design detail that prevents the alteration from happening the easy way, the sleeve must be shortened from the seam that connects it to the shoulder. The sleeve is completely removed, shortened, and reattached. And, of course, the price goes up, too.

Never underestimate the power of a simple alteration to help you look your absolute best. In times of crises, your tailor or seamstress can be your go-to guy or gal to achieve a custom fit. Remember—tailoring is the original makeover. It can take the ordinary, the flawed, and the not quite right and transform them into the exceptional, the polished, and the absolute best. The "before" and "after" magic of good tailoring can go a long way toward refining your wardrobe and your sense of style.

PROPER SLEEVE LENGTH

CHAPTER 9

Taking Inventory

THE ULTIMATE CLOSET CLEANOUT

$Okay,$ $it's$ $time$ to face the music. We all have closets filled with clothes. Some we wear, some we worship, and some we bought during a momentary lapse of reason. Some are pieces we refuse to let go of because they have served us well over the years. Others are still three sizes too small, but, darn it, one day they will rise again! Or will they?

There comes a time in every woman's journey through style when her closet must be overhauled, cleaned out, and refreshed. This is that time.

Your closet should be your arsenal of style, holding only those items you know you're going to wear. It is not a retirement home for things you might wear again someday. We all know that "someday" never comes. The ultimate closet is filled with clothes that suit your body type, consisting of basics, a few specialty pieces that make you feel your best, the right accessories, and some seasonal jackets, coats, and outerwear.

It should also contain two essentials. The first is your "secret weapon" —that sexy, knock-'em-dead piece that you can pull off the hanger on a

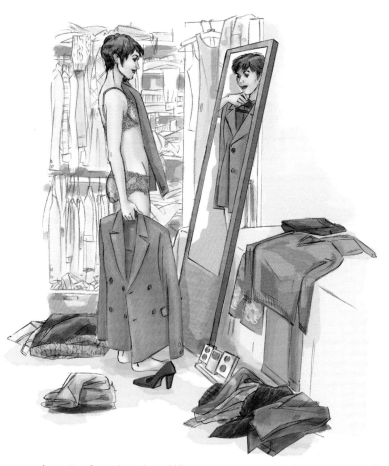

moment's notice for a hot date. When you wear it, you know you've still got it, and it's guaranteed to make him drool. The second is your "tried and true"—the basic item that always looks great no matter what the occasion. It's so perfect, in fact, that you don't even have to look in the mirror when you put it on. If you have these two pieces in your closet, you're as good as gold.

Chances are, much of the stuff tangled in the cobwebs is ready to go, so now you have to come to terms with it and put your wardrobe on a diet. There is work involved here. Gear up; I promise you'll love the end result.

As the seasons change, your clothing needs to change to keep pace, even if you live in a warmer climate. Every six months or so, you should scrutinize your wardrobe and take stock of what you're wearing and what you're not. Your objective is to create two streamlined closets—one that will house your best pieces for the warmer months, and one for the cooler months. If you don't have a second closet to spare, pack a suitcase with the clothes you won't be wearing for six months, and store it away for later.

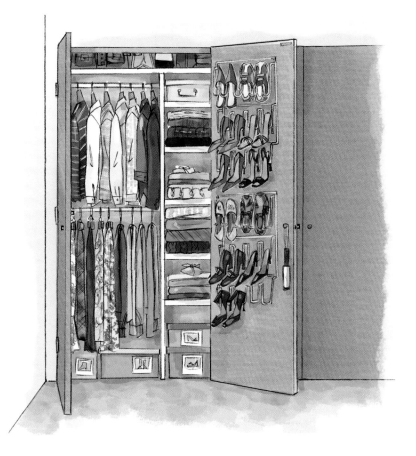

real style secret

THE ARCHIVES

When I buy something I love, I wear it constantly, sometimes to the point where it's played out and tired long before it goes out of style. This habit has resulted in a practical style secret.

I have created a place in my wardrobe called the "archives." It's like a filing cabinet for some of my clothing that needs a break from the rotation of daily dressing. I file these pieces away in the back of my closet in a garment bag, or fold them neatly into a drawer for safekeeping. After several months, I bust them out and put them back into play. I've rediscovered my best pieces and am excited to wear them again.

Every woman should create an archive of her own during a closet clean-out. Down the road, you'll get to shop your closet for your best archived pieces. What's old is new after you've spent some time apart from your favorite clothes

Pick a day you can free up entirely to have a one-on-one with your closet. Start by closing the door to your bedroom, turning on some music, and bringing out a full-length mirror. If you don't have one, pick one up at a discount store for about five bucks. It's definitely a worthwhile investment.

Throw on your best bra and panty so you can really see how the clothes will look, and have a private fashion show. I assure you, yours will be a lot less dramatic and a whole lot more informative than those in New York, Paris, and Milan. Start by trying on the clothes you love to wear, the ones you go to repeatedly, just to make sure they still do it for you. If they look good, check them for stains, holes, snags, and anything that can be improved by tailoring.

Start making piles that reflect your finds. Do some items need hand-washing or dry cleaning? Can some be repaired at home with a needle and thread? Are some of your favorites on their last leg and ready for the donation pile? If so, accept it. Clothing does not last forever, and eventually all good things must come to an end.

Make a pile for cleaning, one for repairs and reinvention by your tailor, one that you'll hand down to your best friend who has always been eyeing that top you're sick of wearing, one you can save for resale or consignment, and one for donation to your local Goodwill or Salvation Army.

Why is it that we become so attached to something only when we think about getting rid of it? Well, certain clothing has a sentimental value. We all have that ratty sweatshirt that has been washed four hundred times—and, yes, it can cheer us up with all of its soft comfort—but we also have to know when to lay it to rest. The best rule to follow is this: If you have not worn something for more than a year, get rid of it.

If it's still in decent shape, try selling it to a resale store. You'll get a small amount of money outright, based on a percentage of the resale price determined by the store. If you have some patience and can wait for payment, you can use the services of a consignment shop. In this case, you get paid a percentage of the selling price *after* the item is sold. Percentages tend to be larger when you sell on consignment—sometimes as high as 60 percent, as opposed to about 35 percent for resale—so it's always the best solution for your high-end items.

A good resale or consignment store will be very picky, carefully choosing what clothing and accessories to accept and what to reject, based on their needs and ability to resell it. If something you've brought in is turned down, at least you tried. Take a drive to your favorite charity and donate it.

If your closet is home to clothes that still have the price tags on them, ask yourself why. Bring yourself back to the moment when you bought each item. Surely you had a reason then, but the fact remains that somehow you never got around to wearing it. Were you caught up in a trend? Was it an impulse buy? Did you buy it in a smaller size to inspire you to lose a few pounds? Did you take on a risk you weren't prepared to face, such as wearing a bright color or a wild pattern?

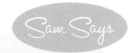
Sam Says

IT'S A WRITE-OFF!

Did you know that some donations could be used as a tax write-off? Talk about good karma. Always get a receipt when you donate old clothing or other personal effects, so you can get the tax deduction *and* a return on your old sense of style. Present that receipt with a smile to your accountant, and your good deed will be rewarded in more ways than one.

REDEEM THOSE TAGS FOR CASH

If you have clothing with price tags on that you know you won't wear, you have four options.

- **ONE:** Try to return it. If you catch your mistake soon enough, take it back to the store and get a refund or exchange it for something you will wear.
- **TWO:** If it's a quality piece, take it to a resale or consignment store that can turn it around for you. Having the original price tag on it may fetch you a better percentage of the price in return, and you can pocket the cash for something new.
- **THREE:** List it on eBay or any other online auction site and start a bidding war on your forgotten fashion.
- **FOUR:** Sell it at a garage sale. Because it's obviously new and never worn, you may be able to command a better price from your prospective buyer.

Whatever the case, you need to figure out if these are mistakes you can learn from, or if they are still-wearable items you need to revisit.

Once you've put some energy into cleaning out your closet, you need to get organized. This is an essential part of the closet-cleanout extravaganza, because, now that you've trimmed down your stock, you must put it all back together in a strategic way.

There is nothing better than opening a closet full of clothes that are neat and under control. It's a proud display of items you know you'll really wear, and getting dressed will be a snap.

You might try separating your tops from your skirts and bottoms, so you'll always know where to look for what you need. Or you can divide your wardrobe into categories, creating sections for office wear, casual clothes, and evening wear. You can also break things down by color and pattern. You may be happy just to have everything on good, matching hangers. Besides looking neat and organized, everything will lie flush against everything else, eliminating clutter and overflow.

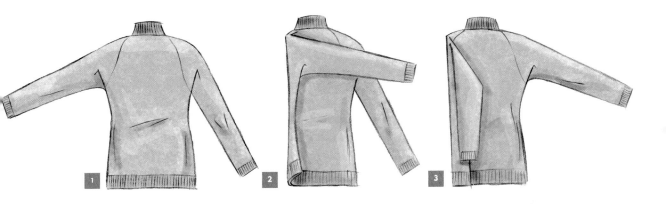

real style secret

ALWAYS FOLD YOUR KNITS

Hanging your knits will stretch them out and cause them to lose their shape. This is also the reason why they should be dried flat after a washing. Always fold your knits and categorize them by weight, separating heavier pieces from lighter ones. You'll maintain their fit and be able to grab the right ones for the right seasons.

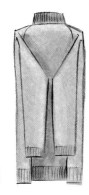

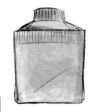

BOX 'EM, DUST 'EM, AND SMILE FOR THE CAMERA

Every time you purchase a new pair of shoes, keep the original box or buy some clear plastic tubs at a discount store as a substitute. Take a Polaroid or digital photo of the shoes, and tape it to the short side of the box. When the boxes are stacked on your closet floor or on a shelf, you can see at a glance what's inside. Your shoes stay organized *and* dust-free, and you'll never forget what you own.

If your space is limited, try using dust bags—those soft felt bags that come with your better shoes. At the very least, your investments are protected and they can be piled neatly on the floor to avoid scuffing or damage. Better still, you have the bags on hand for a quick buff and polish.

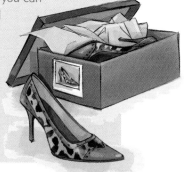

With all your excess clothing out of the way and your closet neatly ordered, you need to direct your attention downward, to the piles of shoes, boots, and sandals collecting dust and dander on the floor. After you weed out the ones that have to go and discover those that can be saved by the cobbler, organize your shoes by color or style and keep them in pairs along the floor or up on a shelf.

When you're organizing your closet, it's smart to take advantage of every available nook and cranny. One place that is often overlooked is your closet door. I buy hanging shoe organizers and large hooks that hang over the tops of doors. I put all my flat sandals in the pockets of the shoe organizer, freeing up space for my everyday shoes. I use the hooks on the doors for everything—to lay out an outfit for the next day, or to hang my clothes temporarily when I come home late and don't feel like returning them to their proper place. Be creative with any free space.

Just one last piece of advice to round things out: Now that you've tidied things up and you realize what your closet might be missing, you may feel the need to fill it back up with items that reflect your new understanding of style. That's fine, but keep this in mind: You started out by getting rid of items that were blah, so make sure your replacement pieces are stellar.

KEEP THAT CLOSET FRESH

• **Cedar**—This natural wood has a fresh, outdoorsy scent that repels moths. Tuck some small cedar blocks against the baseboards of your closet, hang some cedar balls in a breathable bag, or place cedar disks on your hangers.

• **Baking Soda**—Place an opened box of baking soda in a back corner of your closet. It will absorb odors and help regulate moisture that can harbor mold. Vacuuming with baking soda is essential if your closet is carpeted, and should be done once a month.

• **Essential Oils**—Put a few drops on a piece of medical gauze, and tape to the wall or under a shelf. The scent will pass easily through the airy cloth. Try eucalyptus oil for its antibacterial properties. Be sure to keep any oil safely away from your clothing to prevent stains.

• **Sachets**—These breathable bags are filled with potpourri and scented with oil. Place them in your intimates drawer, hang them in your closet, or pack them in a suitcase for your next vacation.

• **Fabric-Softener Sheets**—Toss a sheet or two in each drawer of your dresser or ball some up in a shoe, to keep everything smelling clean and freshly laundered. Just remember to change them every month or so.

CHAPTER 10

Just Looking

MASTERING THE ART OF SHOPPING

It seems only natural that your journey toward real style would eventually lead you to the final step: the shopping trip. *Yes!* Clothes, shoes, accessories—they're all out there waiting for you. Racks and shelves teeming with merchandise, taunting you, inviting you to buy it so you can show off everything you've learned about style. Sorry, girls—not just yet.

I have one little assignment for you—a final exam, if you will: Take all the facts and secrets you've amassed, toss this book in your purse, grab a friend, and **spend the day shopping—*without buying a single thing.***

Yep—you heard me correctly. And no—I haven't lost my mind. This will become perfectly logical once you begin to understand that **a single "just looking" shopping trip will result in the ability to make informed purchases for the rest of your life.**

Think about it for a minute. Stylists know so much about fashion

GET INSPIRED

Go through your favorite magazines and tear out pictures of clothing you think you'd look good in and things you've always wanted to wear but never had the guts to try. You'll basically be compiling a story-board of looks that will inspire you. Then go find similar items in the stores to see if your gut was right.

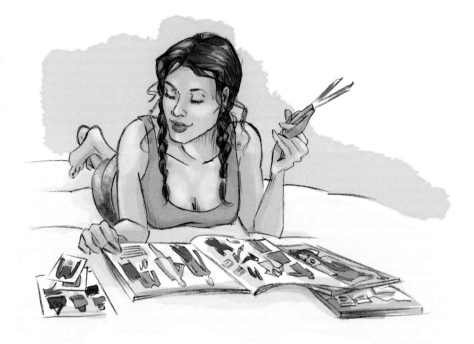

because we are constantly surrounded by stores and clothing. We have the opportunity to play dress-up with our clients over and over again, using these experiences to perfect our talents. Over time, we figure out exactly what shops to hit first and what designer is best matched to a specific personality or body type. After your day of shopping, you can do the same. It's all a game of trial and error, so get ready to play it.

Begin by wandering in and out of the stores in your area, "editing" them to find the ones that offer the clothing and accessories best suited to your body type and emerging sense of style. This means keeping an eye out for cuts, styles, and colors that work, and zipping right past those that don't. After all you've learned in these pages, you'll know immediately when something is on target—and when to take a pass. Bring a friend with you and ask for her honest opinion as you shop.

Remind her, if you have to, that a real pal lets you know if something doesn't look good on you. (I know I would.) She has a perspective you can't buy, so her appraisal is priceless.

An exploratory shopping trip will also help you determine what stores are best for each type of purchase. Like the pros, you'll be creating a network of go-to shops. By using this strategy, you'll learn which shops have the best pants for you . . . which ones offer an extensive collection of event dresses . . . which ones always stock your favorite basics . . . which ones have the finest jewelry, shoes, and bags. So, when you're in the market for a particular item, you'll know precisely where to go to buy it.

Waltz into that expensive store you once found intimidating. Try on everything that catches your eye to see what all the fuss is about. So what if you can't afford to buy so much as a handkerchief? Who cares if the salespeople give you dirty looks when they realize you have no intention of buying anything? You have every right to be there, so let go of your anxiety. It's just a store, after all, and that's what it's there for.

Wear clothes that are easy to take off and put back on, with a good bra and panty underneath, and sandals that you can slip off in a snap. You should not have to struggle to try things on. Shopping is a workout at times, and when you're on a mission, the less you have to hassle with, the better. You'll thank me by the end of the day.

real style secret

WEAR A WHITE TANK TOP TO SHOP

If you don't want to deal with locked fitting rooms, salespeople, and try-on limits, wear a white tank top when you shop. Choose one you're comfortable wearing in public, because you'll be showing it off. It serves as a perfect foundation, and you can try tops on over it without even entering the fitting room.

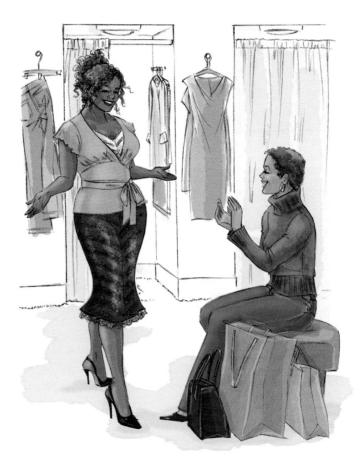

Your day of shopping will entail some work, so take your time. And always try everything on . . . *always*. Even the best shoppers make errors in judgment when they buy without trying—yes, even me. Your assignment is to pay attention to fit and how proportions affect the way your body looks. If something is not quite perfect, ask yourself why. Try to figure out what key elements are missing, or how a tailor could jump in to save the day.

Always choose fit over size. When I was in sales, I encountered many women who would not buy an item because it was a size larger than they thought they were—even when it fit like a glove. I call this vanity shopping, and it doesn't make sense. Why miss out on a great find just because the size doesn't live up to your self-image? You should always buy what works—no matter what the size. If it makes you feel better, cut out the tag to stop that nagging voice in your head that still insists on the size 10 when the 12 is the real winner.

Challenge your comfort zone as often as possible, breaking away from the usual and exploring something new. When an item that you've never dared to try is on the do list for your body type, give it a shot. Remember, this is only a test, so any mistakes you make simply give you an opportunity to learn. Be a kid in a candy store. Take note of everything you love, and create a list—even if it's just in your head.

After a day in the shops, go home and compare your list of great finds with the contents of your closet. Take stock. Is it time to add some excitement to your wardrobe? What do you know now about dressing your best that you didn't know before? And, more important, are you ready to start making some changes? Grab a pen and paper and make your own shopping list. It can be one you add to over time, until you feel it's all in place.

Your list should always begin with a sensible budget. You have to know what you can afford to spend, and stay within those means—or at least close to them. This is part of the reason why I recommend a day of looking without purchasing. It's easy to get caught up in a buying frenzy when you know what to look for. Suddenly everything looks great on you, and you're tempted to buy it all. So it's important to set priorities and limits and buy accordingly.

BE QUEEN FOR A DAY

If you've always wanted to feel like a celebrity on the red carpet but you've never been nominated for an award, do the next-best thing and become queen for a day. Go to that untouchable high-end store and try on a cocktail or evening dress that costs thousands of dollars. Check out all the elements that go into high fashion. Experience the luxury of extraordinary fabrics. See what you look like when you are wearing the best of the best, and then remember that feeling when you find something like it in your own price range. It may surprise you and be just as fabulous.

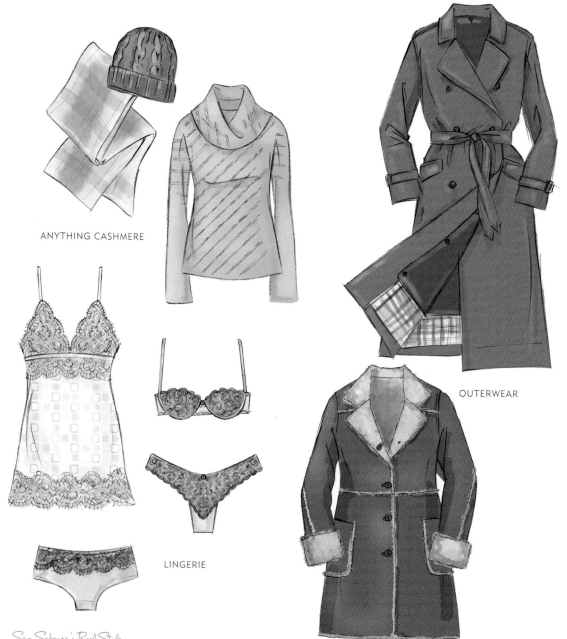

ANYTHING CASHMERE

OUTERWEAR

LINGERIE

PRICY SUMMER SANDALS

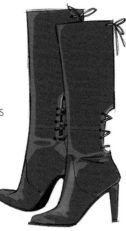

BOOTS

HANDBAGS

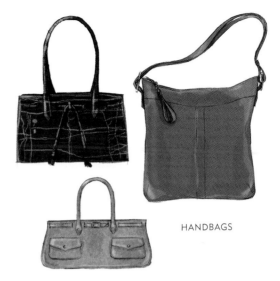

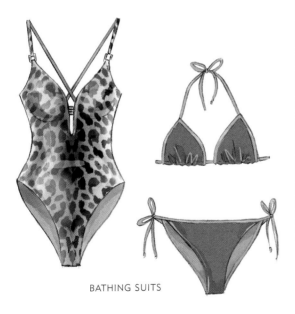

BATHING SUITS

real style secret

THINGS TO BUY WHENEVER YOU FIND THEM ON SALE

- Anything cashmere
- Outerwear
- Pricy summer sandals
- Boots
- Handbags
- Bathing suits
- Lingerie
- Any of the wardrobe basics mentioned in Chapter 3

But remember—just because an item is on sale doesn't mean it's a great find. Fashion disasters can be inexpensive, too. If it doesn't look good enough to buy at full price, don't buy it on sale.

Q I love designer fashions, but I just can't afford them. Is there a way for me to get the look without spending the cash?

A Basically, you have three options here. You can shop the discount stores for designer knockoffs, which will give you the look without the price tag. The quality won't be anywhere near the original, of course, but the trade-off is getting an affordable fashionable style. Try mixing your inexpensive find with something special from your stock to bump it up a notch and give it some value.

Your other choice is to look for the real thing at the outlet stores. This takes more patience and flexibility, but it's definitely worth it if you like the satisfaction of discovering a high-end label on the rack for a steal—and who doesn't?

Finally, check out your local thrift or resale stores, which are bursting with great finds at excellent prices. You might even find some brand-new designer duds with the tags still on for less than half the regular price.

Once you determine exactly what you need to add to your wardrobe, you can go out and start to shop. Try not to stray too far from your list so your budget stays on track, but if you stumble across a great find, grab it. When you're hot, you're hot, so don't mess with the shopping gods if they toss something irresistible in your path.

Enhance your shopping experience by developing a relationship with a salesperson in each of your favorite stores. In fact, you might have one in each department. Over time, these people will become your best assets, because they'll learn what you like and what looks good on you. So, every time you stop by, they'll know exactly what to show you.

Some women are intimidated by salespeople, thinking they have to buy something—whether they like it or not—if the salesperson recommends it. Not

- When you're on a major shopping trip, put everything you like on hold until you're finished looking around, then go back and make your purchases. You'll notice that you buy only the wow pieces, and the rest will seem dull in comparison.
- If something is nagging at you about an item when you try it on, chances are it will bug you even more after you've bought it. Trust your instinct and just say no.
- Always try the size you think you are and the size smaller or larger. You may find that the perfect fit is just a size away.
- When you buy an item of clothing in black, it tends to run smaller than the exact same thing in another color. The overdyeing process required to get a true black often shrinks the garment a bit, so don't be surprised—or disappointed—if you have to go up a size.
- Every time you make a purchase—no matter how big or small, no matter how much you love the item and are sure you'll never return it—keep your sales receipt.
- An expensive purchase can be risky, so always sleep on it. If you wake up and you're still thinking about it the next day, or if you dreamed about it during the night, it's probably meant to be. Go get it with a guilt-free smile.

so. They know that if they delight you time and again, you'll become a regular customer—and that works to their advantage as well as yours.

As you absorb all the new information you've learned about style, you'll find that you'll become a more discriminating shopper. And guess what? That's a pretty good feeling. You'll no longer have the urge to buy something—anything!— just because you're at the mall. Each new purchase you make will be a sensible addition to your wardrobe.

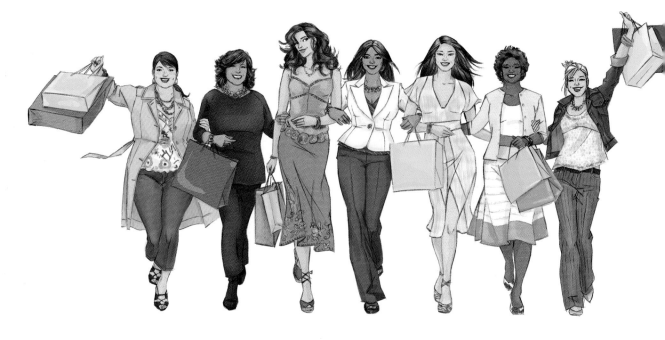

Sam Saboura's Real Style

Okay, ladies, it's time to close the book on style. My work here is done. I've shared as much information as I can . . . I've revealed as many secrets as I know (well, maybe I've kept one or two for another time, another book) . . . and now it's your turn.

So get out there and make it happen. You now have the knowledge and the tools to make a great impression—no matter what you wear, no matter what's on the agenda. Try your best to make the choices that reflect and complement the life you live and the body you're in. And *always* wear what you love.

Above all, don't take style too seriously. It's all in there, but you have to let things evolve over time and happen naturally. Don't run out the door—credit cards in hand, visions of shopping fairies dancing in your head—fixated on revamping your entire wardrobe. Rome wasn't built in a day, and your sense of style won't be, either. Let the changes come gradually, and enjoy every step of the process.

I think the best piece of advice I can leave you with is this: Real style comes from within—not from a fashion magazine, not from a clothing store, not even from a stylist like me, but from you. When you open yourself up to the possibilities, when you least expect it, this whole style thing will become second nature, and you'll make your own brilliant impact.

So what are you waiting for?

index

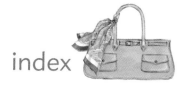

Page numbers in *italic* refer to illustrations.

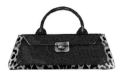

about the author

SAM SABOURA is the breakout star and style host of ABC's hit series *Extreme Makeover*. He has appeared as the fashion and style expert on numerous entertainment, news, and awards programs, and his sought-after style advice regularly appears in national publications.

In addition to dressing the fashion elite of Los Angeles and New York, he is a personal shopper and stylist for celebrities in the film, television, and music industries, where he also works as a freelance wardrobe designer and consultant.

Saboura resides in Los Angeles. Learn more about him and tap into his style tips at samsaboura.com.